Neurology and
Clinical Neuroanatomy
on the move

Neurology and Clinical Neuroanatomy
on the move

Authors: Matthew Tate,
Johnathan Cooper-Knock,
Zoe Hunter and Elizabeth Wood
Editorial Advisor: Daniel J. Blackburn
Series Editors: Rory Mackinnon, Sally Keat,
Thomas Locke and Andrew Walker

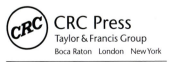

CRC Press
Taylor & Francis Group
Boca Raton   London   New York

CRC Press is an imprint of the
Taylor & Francis Group, an **informa** business

CRC Press
Taylor & Francis Group
6000 Broken Sound Parkway NW, Suite 300
Boca Raton, FL 33487-2742

© 2015 by Matthew Tate, Johnathan Cooper-Knock, Zoe Hunter, and Elizabeth Wood.
CRC Press is an imprint of Taylor & Francis Group, an Informa business

No claim to original U.S. Government works

Printed and bound in India by Replika Press Pvt. Ltd.

Printed on acid-free paper
Version Date: 20140911

International Standard Book Number-13: 978-1-4441-3832-0 (Pack - Book and Ebook)

Library of Congress Cataloging-in-Publication Data

Tate, Matthew, 1987- author.
　　Neurology and clinical neuroanatomy on the move / Matthew Tate, Johnathan Cooper-Knock, Zoe Hunter, and Elizabeth Wood.
　　　p. ; cm. -- (Medicine on the move)
　　Includes index.
　　ISBN 978-1-4441-3832-0 (hardcover : alk. paper)
　　I. Cooper-Knock, Johnathan, 1982- author. II. Hunter, Zoe, 1985- author. III. Wood, Elizabeth, 1986- author. IV. Title. V. Series: Medicine on the move (CRC Press)
　　[DNLM: 1. Nervous System Diseases--Examination Questions. 2. Nervous System--anatomy & histology--Examination Questions. WL 18.2]

RC343.5
616.80076--dc23
2013035959

Visit the Taylor & Francis Web site at
http://www.taylorandfrancis.com

and the CRC Press Web site at
http://www.crcpress.com

Contents

Preface

Do you find Neurology and Neuroanatomy complicated and confusing? Do you struggle to grasp the basics and find core texts difficult to understand? Whether you are preparing for a Neurology rotation or an exam, this revision guide will help you. Written by junior doctors and encompassing flow charts, colourful diagrams, summary tables and key fact boxes – whatever your learning style, you will find this resource informative, easy to read and, we hope, that a once feared topic will become one in which you feel confident and competent.

AUTHORS

Matthew Tate MBChB (Hons) DTM&H – Core Medical Trainee Year 1, Hammersmith Hospital, Imperial College Healthcare NHS Trust, UK

Johnathan Cooper-Knock BMBCh MRCP – Clinical Research Fellow, Sheffield Institute for Translational Neuroscience (SITraN), Sheffield, UK

Zoe Hunter MBChB – GP Trainee Year 3, Tameside and Glossop, North Western Deanery, UK

Elizabeth Wood BMedSci (Hons) MBChB DTM&H DMCC – SHO Emergency Medicine, Hawkes Bay Hospital, Hastings, New Zealand

EDITORIAL ADVISOR

Daniel Blackburn BSc MBChB PhD – Consultant Neurologist, Royal Hallamshire Hospital, Sheffield, UK

EDITOR-IN-CHIEF

Rory Mackinnon MBChB BSc (Hons) – GP Trainee Year 3, The Sele Medical Practice, Hexham, Northumberland, UK

SERIES EDITORS

Sally Keat BMedSci (Hons) MBChB – Core Medical Trainee Year 1, Newham Hospital, London, UK

Thomas Locke BSc MBChB, DTM&H, Core Medical Trainee Year 1, Charing Cross Hospital, London, UK

Andrew M.N. Walker BMedSci MBChB MRCP (London) – BHF Clinical Research Fellow and Honorary Specialist Registrar in Cardiology, Leeds Teaching Hospitals NHS Trust, UK

Acknowledgements

The authors would like to thank the following people for their contribution towards the production of this book:

Professor Pamela Shaw
  Neurology Consultant, Royal Hallamshire Hospital, Sheffield, UK
Dr Oliver Bandmann
  Neurology Consultant, Royal Hallamshire Hospital, Sheffield, UK
Dr Tim Hodgson
  Neuroradiology Consultant, Royal Hallamshire Hospital, Sheffield, UK
Mr John Rochester
  Head of Medical Teaching Unit, University of Sheffield Medical School, UK

List of abbreviations

- 3,4-DAP: 3,4-diaminopyridine
- $5HT_1$: serotonin
- ACA: anterior cerebral artery
- ACE: angiotensin converting enzyme
- AChR: acetylcholine receptor
- ACTH: adrenocorticotrophic hormone
- AD: Alzheimer's disease
- ADEM: acute disseminated encephalomyelitis
- ADPCKD: autosomal dominant polycystic kidney disease
- AF: atrial fibrillation
- AIDP: acute inflammatory demyelinating polyradiculoneuropathy
- AIDS: acquired immune deficiency syndrome
- AION: anterior ischaemic optic neuropathy
- AIP: acute intermittent porphyria
- ALS: amyotrophic lateral sclerosis
- AMAN: acute motor axonal neuropathy
- ANA: anti-nuclear antibody
- ANCA: anti-neutrophil cytoplasmic antibody
- ATPase: adenosine triphosphatase
- AVM: arteriovenous malformation
- AZT: zidovudine
- BiPAP: bi-level positive airway pressure
- BMD: Becker muscular dystrophy
- BPPV: benign paroxysmal positional vertigo
- CADASIL: cerebral autosomal dominant angiopathy and stroke ischemic leucodystrophy
- cANCA: cytoplasmic anti-neutrophil cytoplasmic antibody
- CBD: corticobasal degeneration
- CIDP: chronic inflammatory demyelinating polyneuropathy
- CJD: Creutzfeld–Jakob disease
- CMV: cytomegalovirus
- CNS: central nervous system
- COMT: catechol-o-methyltransferase
- CPH: chronic paroxysmal hemicrania
- CPK: creatinine phosphokinase
- CRAg: cryptococcal antigen
- CRP: C-reactive protein
- CSF: cerebrospinal fluid
- CT: computed tomography

- DANISH: dysdiadochokinesis, ataxia, nystagmus, intention tremor, scanning speech, hypotonia
- DLB: dementia with Lewy bodies
- DMD: Duchenne muscular dystrophy
- *DMPK*: myotonic dystrophy protein kinase (gene)
- DWI: diffusion-weighted imaging
- EBV: Epstein–Barr virus
- ECG: electrocardiography
- ED: emergency department
- EDH: extradural haematoma
- EEG: electroencephalography
- EMG: electromyogram
- ESR: erythrocyte sedimentation rate
- FSH: follicle-stimulating hormone
- FVC: forced vital capacity
- GBS: Guillain–Barré syndrome
- GCA: giant cell arteritis
- GCS: Glasgow Coma Scale
- GI: gastrointestinal
- GP: general practitioner
- GPI: general paresis of the insane
- HAART: highly active antiretroviral therapy
- HbA1$_C$: glycosylated haemoglobin
- HD: Huntington's disease
- HDU: high-dependency unit
- HIV: human immunodeficiency virus
- HLA: human leukocyte antigen
- HMSN: hereditary motor and sensory neuropathy
- HONK: hyperosmotic non-ketotic (coma)
- HSV: herpes simplex virus
- ICP: intracranial pressure
- IDE: idiopathic generalised epilepsy
- IIH: idiopathic intracranial hypertension
- IM: intramuscular
- INO: internuclear ophthalmoplegia
- IPD: idiopathic Parkinson's disease
- ITU: intensive therapy unit
- IV: intravenous
- IVDU: intravenous drug user
- IVIG: intravenous immunoglobulin
- LEMS: Lambert–Eaton myasthenic syndrome
- LFT: liver function test
- LGN: lateral geniculate nucleus

- LH: luteinizing hormone
- LMN: lower motor neuron
- LOAF: lumbricals, opponens pollicis, abductor pollicis brevis and flexor pollicis brevis
- LOLA: L-ornithine and L-aspartate
- LP: lumbar puncture
- MAO-B: monoamine oxidase B
- MCA: middle cerebral artery
- MCI: mild cognitive impairment
- MCV: mean corpuscular volume
- MDT: multidisciplinary team
- MEN: multiple endocrine neoplasia
- MG: myasthenia gravis
- MLF: medial longitudinal fasciculus
- MMSE: Mini-Mental State Examination
- MND: motor neuron disease
- MPTP: methylphenyltetrahydropyridine
- MRA: magnetic resonance angiography
- MRI: magnetic resonance imaging
- MRV: magnetic resonance venography
- MS: multiple sclerosis
- MSA: multiple system atrophy
- MuSK: muscle-specific tyrosine kinase
- NCS: nerve conduction studies
- NF: neurofibromatosis
- NIV: non-invasive intermittent ventilation
- NMDA: N-methyl-D-aspartate
- NMJ: neuromuscular junction
- NMO: neuromyelitis optica
- NSE: neuron-specific enolase
- ON: optic neuropathy
- PACS: partial anterior circulation stroke
- pANCA: perinuclear anti-neutrophil cytoplasmic antibody
- PCR: polymerase chain reaction
- PCT: porphyria cunea tarda
- PDD: Parkinson's disease-associated dementia
- PET: positive emission tomography
- PICA: posterior inferior cerebellar artery
- PLS: primary lateral sclerosis
- PMA: progressive muscular atrophy
- PML: progressive multifocal leucoencephalopathy
- PMR: polymyalgia rheumatica
- PNS: peripheral nervous system

- PoCS: posterior circulation stroke
- PPMS: primary progressive multiple sclerosis
- PSP: progressive supranuclear palsy
- QDS: four times daily
- RAPD: relative afferent pupillary defect
- REM: rapid eye movement
- RRMS: relapsing-remitting multiple sclerosis
- SACD: subacute combined degeneration (of the spinal cord)
- SAH: subarachnoid haemorrhage
- SCA: spinocerebellar ataxias
- SCLC: small cell lung cancer
- SDH: subdural haematoma
- SIADH: syndrome of inappropriate anti-diuretic hormone secretion
- SLE: systemic lupus erythematosus
- SPECT: single-photon emission computed tomography
- SUDEP: sudden unexpected death in epilepsy
- SSPE: subacute sclerosing panencephalitis
- TACS: total anterior circulation stroke
- TB: tuberculosis
- TIA: transient ischaemic attack
- T-LOC: transient loss of consciousness
- TNFα: tumour necrosis factor-alpha
- TPHA: *Treponema pallidum* haemagglutination
- TSC1: tuberous sclerosis gene 1
- TSC2: tuberous sclerosis gene 2
- TSH: thyroid-stimulating hormone
- UMN: upper motor neuron
- VA: ventriculoatrial
- vCJD: new variant Creutzfeld–Jakob disease
- VDRL: venereal disease research laboratory (test)
- VEP: visual evoked potential
- VGKC: voltage gated potassium channel
- VLA-4: very late antigen-4
- VP: ventriculoperitoneal
- VZV: varicella zoster virus
- *ZNF9*: zinc finger protein 9 (gene)

An explanation of the text

The book is divided into four parts: Clinical neurology; Neurological zones; Neurological disorders; and Self-assessment. We have used bullet points to keep the text concise and supplemented this with a range of diagrams, pictures and MICRO-boxes (explained in the following material).

Where possible, we have endeavoured to include treatment options for each condition. Nevertheless, drug sensitivities and clinical practices are constantly under review, so always check your local guidelines for up-to-date information.

> ## MICRO-facts
> These boxes expand on the text and contain clinically relevant facts and memorable summaries of the essential information.

> **MICRO-print**
> These boxes contain additional information to the text that may interest certain readers but is not essential for everybody to learn.

> **MICRO-case**
> These boxes contain clinical cases relevant to the text and include a number of summary bullet points to highlight the key learning objectives.

> **MICRO-reference**
> These boxes contain references to important clinical research and national guidance.

Part **1**

Clinical neurology

1 Neurological symptoms and signs

1.1 SYMPTOMS AND SIGNS FLOW CHARTS

- The flow charts and table on the following pages are designed to allow the rapid generation of differential diagnoses for some of the common neurological presenting symptoms and signs.
    - Causes of altered facial expression (see **Fig. 1.1**)
    - Causes of limb weakness (see **Fig. 1.2**)
    - Causes of weakness by location of lesion and speed of onset (see **Table 1.1**)
    - Causes of sensory loss (see **Fig. 1.3**)
    - Causes of ptosis (see **Fig. 1.4**)
    - Causes of pupillary abnormalities (see **Fig. 1.5**)
    - Causes of visual loss (see **Fig. 1.6**)
- They may also be used 'backwards' (i.e. working bottom to top) to understand the group of symptoms and signs that are suggestive of a particular condition or of disease affecting a particular anatomical zone.

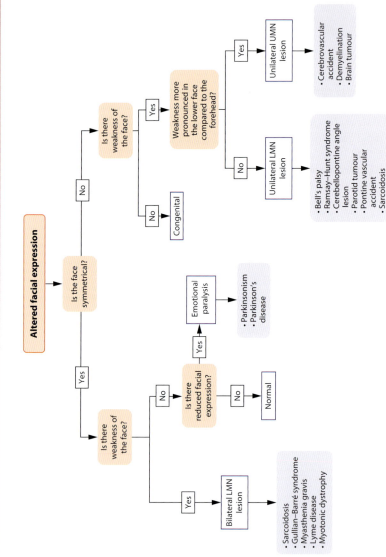

Fig. 1.1 Causes of altered facial expression.

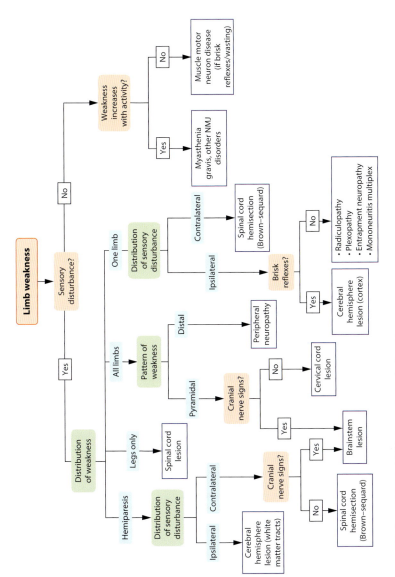

Fig. 1.2 Causes of limb weakness. NMJ, neuromuscular junction.

Table 1.1 Causes of weakness by location of lesion and speed of onset

	ACUTE (MINUTES)	SUBACUTE (HOURS TO DAYS)	CHRONIC (WEEKS TO YEARS)
Cerebral hemisphere	• Stroke or transient ischaemic attack (TIA) • Trauma	• Multiple sclerosis • Abscess/infection (meningitis and encephalitis)	• Neurodegeneration • Tumour
Brainstem	• Stroke • Trauma	• Multiple sclerosis	• Tumour
Spinal cord	• Stroke • Trauma	• Multiple sclerosis • Transverse myelitis • Infection (e.g. epidural abscess) • Cord compression (e.g. disc prolapse)	• Tumour • Syringomyelia • Toxic/metabolic degeneration • Motor neuron disease
Nerve root	• Trauma	• Infection	• Tumour • Disc prolapse
Peripheral nerve	• Infarction • Trauma	• Guillain–Barré syndrome • Entrapment neuropathy • Infective/ inflammatory mononeuropathy	• Toxic/metabolic/ endocrine neuropathy
Neuromuscular junction			• Myasthenia gravis • Lambert–Eaton myasthenic syndrome (LEMS)
Muscle		• Necrotising myopathy	• Polymyositis/ dermatomyositis • Muscular dystrophy • Myotonic dystrophy

Clinical neurology

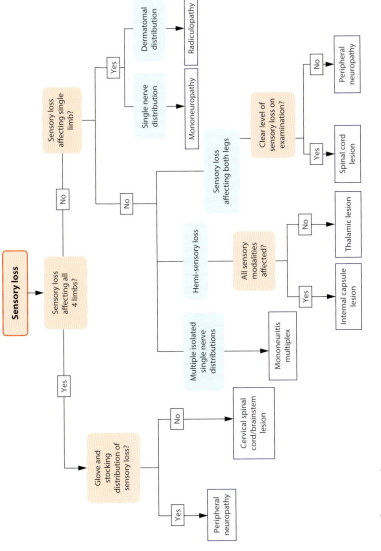

Fig. 1.3 Causes of sensory loss.

Clinical neurology

Clinical neurology

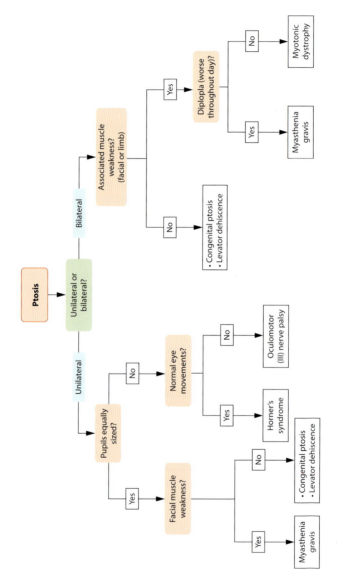

Fig. 1.4 Causes of ptosis.

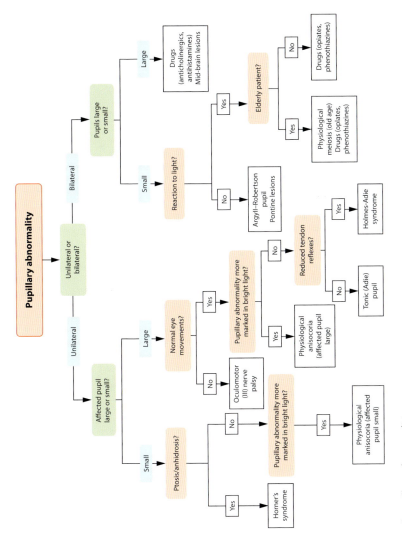

Fig. 1.5 Causes of pupillary abnormalities.

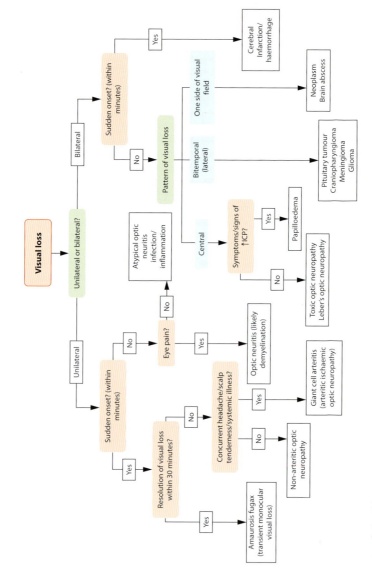

Fig. 1.6 Causes of visual loss.

1.2 MOVEMENT DISORDERS

- Disorders of movement may feature positive phenomena (tremor) or negative phenomena (akinesia).
- It is notable that many movement disorders result from pathology within the basal ganglia.
  - The basal ganglia are involved in the internal generation ('I'm going to walk') of voluntary movement as opposed to externally cued movement like dancing to music (sometimes preserved in parkinsonism).
  - Pathology can lead to **bradykinesia** (slow movements of reduced amplitude) as in Parkinson's disease or **dyskinesia** (excess movement), which can take a variety of forms described in the following material.
- The various symptoms of movement disorders can be categorized as follows: tremor, chorea, hemiballismus, dystonia, athetosis, tic, myoclonus, akathisia and asterixis.

TREMOR

- Involuntary, rhythmic, oscillatory muscle movement involving one or more parts of the body.
- Types of tremor **(see Table 1.2)**.

CHOREA

- Movements are involuntary, brief, irregular, random and unpredictable.
- The patient is often not aware of them.
- These movements can improve with drugs that block **dopaminergic** activity within the basal ganglia.
- **Causes** of chorea include:
  - neuroleptic drugs;
  - Huntington's disease;
  - Sydenham's chorea (rare);
  - stroke (hemi-chorea).

HEMIBALLISMUS

- Uncontrolled violent movements affecting the proximal muscles of one side of the body.
- Worse on action and disappear during sleep.
- Results from pathology affecting the contralateral basal ganglia, particularly the subthalamic nucleus and its connections, including:
  - stroke;
  - multiple sclerosis;
  - traumatic brain injury.

Table 1.2 **Types of tremor**

TREMOR	FEATURES	CAUSES
Parkinsonian	• Occurs at rest and while walking. • Classically **'pill-rolling'** tremor of the **hand(s)**. • **Asymmetrical**: Onset is typically unilateral with progression to involve the other side. • Tremor **amplitude may be increased by a stressor,** such as asking the patient to perform serial-7 subtractions. • Associated with other features of **Parkinsonism.**	• **Parkinson's disease** • Drug induced (e.g. antipsychotics like chlorpromazine, haloperidol) • Wilson's disease (rare but important)
Essential	• Postural: occurs on holding the arms out. • Typically **symmetrical tremor** of the **hands**. • May be ameliorated by **alcohol.** • May be mild and non-progressive. • **Not** usually associated with other symptomatology.	• 50% of cases likely due to as-yet-unidentified autosomal dominant **mutation**(s)
Cerebellar	• Occurs at the **end of a purposeful movement, such as touching a target**. • Associated with other features of **cerebellar disease, such as nystagmus and dysarthria.** • Unilateral or bilateral depending on the nature of the cerebellar pathology; occurs **ipsilateral to cerebellar disease.**	• Multiple sclerosis • Wernicke's encephalopathy • Spinocerebellar ataxias (rare) • Posterior circulation stroke
Physiological	• Small-amplitude postural tremor in **normal** individuals when anxious or after exercise.	Factors that may **enhance** a physiological tremor: • Hyperthyroidism • Hypoglycaemia • Drugs (e.g. beta-agonists) • Alcohol withdrawal

DYSTONIA

- Co-contraction of antagonistic muscles results in abnormal posture and/or twisting movements. It may be **focal**, affecting only one or two areas of the body, or **generalised**.
- **Causes** of dystonia include:
  - neuroleptic drugs;
  - genetics;
  - stroke;
  - traumatic brain injury;
  - Wilson's disease.

ATHETOSIS

- Slow and repetitive involuntary writhing movements that can affect any part of the body, but most commonly the fingers, toes and face.
  - Athetosis is a dystonic movement, and there is usually a postural disturbance.
  - Most commonly, athetosis is associated with cerebral palsy.

TIC

- Tics are brief, repetitive stereotyped movements often preceded by a sensation of having to do it (like a sneeze).
- Attempts to voluntarily suppress tics often make them worse.
- They may be distractible.
- **Causes** of tics include:
  - genetics:
    - simple tics;
    - complex tics (Gilles de la Tourette syndrome).

MYOCLONUS

- Myoclonic jerks are sudden and brief involuntary contractions of a muscle group, resulting in limb jerking.
- Myoclonus results from lesions affecting the cortex, subcortex and spinal cord.
- **Causes** of myoclonus include:
  - multiple sclerosis;
  - Creutzfeldt–Jakob disease;
  - epilepsy (juvenile myoclonic epilepsy, other childhood epilepsies);
  - Alzheimer's disease;
  - subacute sclerosing panencephalitis (SSPE; a long-term complication of measles infection).

AKATHISIA

- Akathisia is characterised by significant motor restlessness, which may result in an inability to lie or sit still. Sleeping may also become problematic.

Clinical neurology

- **Causes** of akathisia are:
  - phenothiazines (e.g. chlorpromazine);
  - Parkinson's disease;
  - restless leg syndrome.

ASTERIXIS

- **Asterixis** consists of irregular jerky extension and flexion movements at the wrist and metacarpophalangeal joints. It is more commonly known as the 'flapping tremor' and more easily elicited with the arms outstretched and the hands in dorsiflexion.
  - Occurs as a result of loss of **proprioception** input to the reticular formation in the brainstem.
- Asterixis is most often associated with **liver failure** (see Section 20.2).
  - Other causes include:
    - cardiac failure;
    - respiratory failure;
    - renal failure;
    - hypoglycaemia;
    - barbiturate intoxication (e.g. phenobarbitol).

1.3 BULBAR SYMPTOMS

- A group of symptoms that result from motor dysfunction of the muscles innervated by the lower cranial nerves (IX, X, XI, XII; see Section 6.2).

DYSARTHRIA

- Dysarthria is the abnormal speech resulting from impaired motor function.
- Types of dysarthria are shown in **Table 1.3**.

DYSPHONIA

- Related to dysfunction of the vocal chords within the larynx. The voice becomes husky in nature, and patients classically present with a 'bovine cough'.
- Caused by pathology of the larynx, either a structural lesion or a paralysis related to a recurrent laryngeal nerve palsy (e.g. in lung cancer).

DYSPHAGIA

- Dysphagia is difficulty **swallowing** (of food and/or liquid).
  - Structural causes of dysphagia affecting the pharynx typically impair swallowing of liquids:
    - pharyngeal pouch;
    - neoplasm.

Table 1.3 **Types of dysarthria**

	FEATURES	PATHOPHYSIOLOGY	CAUSES
Spastic	Slurred, forced and effortful speech; slow tongue movements with a brisk jaw jerk	• Bilateral UMN weakness • Damage to pyramidal tract	• Pseudobulbar palsy • Motor neuron disease
Extrapyramidal (*not* really dysarthria)	Rapid monotonous speech without rhythm, sentences start and stop abruptly	• Bilateral or unilateral damage to the LMN • Basal ganglia dysfunction	• Parkinsonism • Parkinson's disease • Huntington's disease
Cerebellar	Slurred speech with an irregular rhythm	• Damage to the cerebellum	• Alcohol intoxication • Demyelination • Phenytoin toxicity • Cerebellum stroke

LMN, lower motor neuron; UMN, upper motor neuron.

- Structural causes affecting the oesophagus typically impair swallowing of solids:
  - oesophageal stricture;
  - neoplasm;
  - achalasia;
  - scleroderma.
- Neuromuscular disease causing dysphagia will cause dysphagia to both solids and liquids equally:
  - myasthenia gravis;
  - bulbar or pseudobulbar palsy (see Table 6.2).

1.4 HEARING LOSS

- Hearing loss is either **conductive** or **sensorineural**.
- **Conductive** hearing loss results from reduced conduction of sound waves anywhere from the outer ear, through the tympanic membrane and ossicles to the cochlea.
  - Causes include:
    - wax/foreign body;
    - tympanic membrane perforation;

      – otitis media;
      – otosclerosis.
- **Sensorineural** hearing loss results from pathology of the organ of Corti in the inner ear or the afferent neural pathway.
  - It represents an inability to transduce sound into a neural signal and transmit it to higher centres in the cortex.
  - Causes include:
    - congenital aplasia of the cochlea;
    - presbycusis (age-related hearing loss);
    - cholesteatoma;
    - acoustic neuroma;
    - drugs (e.g. aminoglycosides);
    - Meniere's disease;
    - infection (e.g. mumps, meningitis).

MICRO-facts

- It is possible to differentiate between **conductive** and **sensorineural** hearing loss using **Weber's** and **Rinne's** tests:
  - **Weber's** test consists of holding a tuning fork in contact with the forehead. The sound will be louder in the affected ear in conductive hearing loss and louder in the unaffected ear in sensorineural hearing loss.
  - **Rinne's** test consists of holding a tuning fork in the air around the ear and in contact with the mastoid process. In conductive hearing loss, the sound will be louder via bone conduction; in sensorineural hearing loss, utilising bone conduction will not improve the hearing loss.

1.5 ABNORMALITIES OF EYE MOVEMENT

STRABISMUS

- **Strabismus** occurs when the visual axis of each eye are not directed simultaneously at the same object.
- It may occur due to a **problem in the vision through one eye** (usually a refractive error).
  - The brain compensates for this by reducing dependence on the affected eye and stopping the eyes working together in unison.
  - In this case, both eyes have the full range of movement, which may be demonstrated by assessing them independently, and a patient will **not** have symptomatic **diplopia**. This is the commonly described 'squint'.

- Alternatively, a strabismus may be caused by a **paralysis** of one or more movements of either eye due to pathology of the extraoccular muscles or the efferent neural pathways.
  - In paralytic strabismus, the range of movement of the eye(s) is impaired, and the patient will complain of **diplopia**.
  - Causes include:
    - myopathy (e.g. chronic progressive external ophthalmoplegia);
    - myasthenia gravis;
    - cranial nerve lesions, including peripheral neuropathy (see Section 6.2);
    - brainstem pathology (e.g. neoplasm or stroke).

NYSTAGMUS

- Nystagmus is a repetitive and involuntary oscillation of the eyes. A few beats of nystagmus at the extremities of gaze is normal, but sustained nystagmus is always pathological.
- Nystagmus may result from pathology in a number of different regions:
  - **Peripheral vestibular** disease (see Chapter 7) will cause horizontal nystagmus associated with other symptoms, such as vertigo.
  - **Cerebellar** disease (see Section 6.5) will cause nystagmus that is horizontal and gaze evoked. In unilateral cerebellar disease, nystagmus will typically be exhibited on gaze towards the side of the lesion and will have a fast phase towards that same side. Patients will also exhibit other features of cerebellar disease.
  - **Brainstem** pathology may cause nystagmus in any direction, for example, an **Arnold–Chiari malformation** (see Section 6.5).
- **Drugs** may cause nystagmus (e.g. **lithium** and **carbamazepine**).

1.6 ABNORMAL GAIT

Gait abnormalities

	DESCRIPTION	PATHOPHYSIOLOGY	COMMON CAUSES
Cerebellar ataxia	Patients have a wide-based gait, slow and less steady when turning.	Cerebellar pathology	• Drugs • Multiple sclerosis • Stroke

(*Continued*)

Clinical neurology

Gait abnormalities (*Continued*)

	DESCRIPTION	PATHOPHYSIOLOGY	COMMON CAUSES
Hemiparetic gait	Patients will swing one leg outwards while walking; the arm on the same side may be held in a flexed position.	Contralateral upper motor neuron lesion causing contralateral pyramidal pattern weakness	• Stroke • Multiple sclerosis
Marche à petits pas gait	The patient will have small paces but normal posture and arm swing.	Due to diffuse cortical dysfunction	• Stroke
Parkinsonian gait	Patients will have a stooped posture and reduced arm swing with a small paced gait.	Due to basal ganglia dysfunction	• Parkinson's disease • Antipsychotic medication
Scissoring gait	Patients have bilateral excessive adduction of the hip during leg swing.	Due to a spastic paraparesis	• Cerebral palsy • Multiple sclerosis • Spinal cord compression
Sensory ataxia	Similar to cerebellar ataxia but patients will have a positive Romberg's test.	Indicates a loss of joint position sense	• Peripheral neuropathy • Loss of posterior column function
Steppage gait (foot drop)	Patients are unable to dorsiflex the foot and will therefore have a high-stepping gait		• Common peroneal nerve injury • L5 radiculopathy • Peripheral neuropathy • Motor neuron disease
Waddling gait	The patient's pelvis will rotate on walking.	Due to proximal muscle weakness	• Proximal myopathy • Congenital dislocation of the hip

2 Neurological history and examination

2.1 THE NEUROLOGICAL HISTORY

HISTORY OF PRESENTING COMPLAINT

- How long did the symptoms last? Are they constant or intermittent? Do they occur at certain times of the day/week/month?
  - The chronicity of symptoms is especially vital in making a clinical diagnosis in neurology, as many pathological processes can produce similar symptoms and signs – often the speed of onset suggests a particular disease process (see **Table 2.1**).
- Ask about the character of the symptoms, including their location and distribution.
- Are the symptoms stable/improved/worsening?
- Are there any precipitating, exacerbating or relieving factors?
  - What was the patient doing when the symptoms occurred (e.g. posture related, exercising, sleeping, coughing)?
- Any associated symptoms?
- Ask general questions about other possible neurological dysfunction:
  - headache;
  - fits or faints;
  - dizziness or vertigo;
  - disturbance in vision (e.g. double vision, blurred vision or photophobia);
  - change in hearing or smell;

Table 2.1 **Speed of onset of neurological symptoms**

SPEED OF ONSET OF NEUROLOGICAL SYMPTOMS	CAUSE OF SYMPTOMS
Acute (minutes to hours)	Vascular source
Subacute (days to weeks)	Inflammation, infection or metabolic source
Chronic (months to years)	Neurodegeneration or neoplastic source

- difficulty walking;
- weakness in limbs;
- involuntary movements or tremor;
- history of falls;
- sensory symptoms;
- disturbance of sphincter function (bowels, bladder, sexual function);
- speech/language/swallowing disturbance (e.g. dysarthria/dysphasia);
- difficulties with memory or other cognitive function.

PAST MEDICAL HISTORY

- Aside from taking a full history of previous medical conditions, several points may be significant:
  - Migraine can occur at any age, but very commonly patients had a headache as a teenager that was migrainous.
  - Febrile seizure, if prolonged and requiring hospital admission, increases risk of focal epilepsy.
  - Major head trauma (requiring neurosurgery) and childhood meningitis may also increase the risk of focal epilepsy.

Drug history

- Many drugs can have toxic effects on the nervous system:
  - peripheral neuropathies (alcohol, chemotherapeutics, anti-retrovirals);
  - cerebellar syndrome (alcohol, phenytoin, carbamazepine).

Social history

- Use of recreational drugs is important. Cocaine can cause young-onset stroke.

Collateral history

- It is essential to take a collateral history from a close relative or associate, especially for cognitive impairment, seizures or altered consciousness.

2.2 THE NEUROLOGICAL EXAMINATION

CRANIAL NERVES

- A general examination, looking for scars, ptosis, proptosis, facial asymmetry or pupil inequality, is important.

Olfactory nerve (I)

- Olfaction can be tested through each nostril with strong, recognisable smells (e.g. peppermint). This is rarely done.

Optic nerve (II)

- **Visual inattention**: Hold your fingers in the periphery of the visual field and move your fingertips on each side consecutively and then simultaneously; ask the patient to report which hand is moving. If there is inattention (non-dominant parietal lobe lesion), the patient will detect isolated movement on both sides but will ignore one side when movement is in both simultaneously.

- **Visual acuity**: Test each eye separately. Ideally, use a **Snellen chart**.
  - If a patient usually wears glasses, the patient's acuity should be assessed while wearing them.
  - If the patient is unable to see the top line at 1 m, check if the patient can count fingers, see hand movements or discriminate between the presence and absence of a light.
- **Colour vision**:
  - Ask the patient to look at a bright yellow sharps bin and say if it is equally bright in either eye (colour desaturation – seen in optic neuritis).
  - Formal colour vision testing with Ishihara plates can be performed if necessary.
- **Accommodation**:
  - Ask the patient to focus on a distant object and then your finger held 30 cm in front of his or her nose. Normal accommodation response involves convergence of the eyes and bilateral simultaneous constriction of both pupils.
- **Visual fields**: May be examined crudely at the bedside.
  - **Peripheral**: Sit about 1 m away from the patient with your eyes at the same horizontal level. Cover one of the patient's eyes and close your eye that is opposite. Slowly move your finger into the upper and lower quadrants of the patient's temporal fields. Examine the patient's nasal field using the same technique.
  - **Central**: Ask the patient to cover one eye and look directly at you; ask if any of your face is missing.
- **Pupil responses to light**:
  - Assess the size and shape of pupils; ask patient to look straight ahead and shine a pen torch into the pupil. Look for the direct (ipsilateral) and consensual (contralateral) responses.
  - **Swinging torch test**: Used to assess for a **relative afferent pupillary defect** (damage to one optic nerve relative to the other).
    - Move the torch in an arc from pupil to pupil, pausing for 3 seconds on each eye. When the light is shone on the normal side, a normal direct and consensual response occurs.
    - When the light is shone on the abnormal side, both pupils paradoxically dilate due to relaxation of the pupillary muscles and an impaired direct response. This demonstrates slowed conduction in the optic nerve.
- **Fundoscopy**: Ask the patient to focus on a distant target in dimmed light.
  - First bring the red reflex into focus from a distance of around 10 cm.

- Move closer to the patient's head to find a retinal vessel, then follow it back to the optic disc.
- Assess the cupping, contour and colour of the optic disc and its margins.
- The arteries are a deeper red and narrower than the veins. Look for retinal vein pulsation (normally present in approximately 80% of individuals; difficult to observe), a sign of normal intracranial pressure.
- Examine the rest of the retina, looking for haemorrhages, discolouration and white patches of exudate.
- Ask patient to look at the light of the ophthalmoscope, which brings the macula into view.

Oculomotor (III), trochlear (IV) and abducens (VI) nerves

- Observe for ptosis.
- **Eye movements**:
  - Test movements in all directions by asking the patient to hold his or her head still and follow the movement of your finger. Visual pursuit should be smooth. Observe for abnormal movements or nystagmus. Ask the patient to report any pain or double vision.

Trigeminal nerve (V)

- **Sensation**: Test using cotton wool over the forehead, medial aspects of cheeks and the chin (corresponds to the three divisions of the trigeminal nerve).
- **Motor**:
  - Ask the patient to clench his or her teeth and palpate the patient's masseters and temporalis. Ask the patient to open the jaw against resistance (pterygoids). A unilateral lesion will cause the jaw to deviate towards the side of the lesion as the mouth is opened.
- **Corneal reflex**: Lightly touch the cornea with a wisp of cotton wool brought in from the side. If the reflex is intact, both eyes will blink. The sensory component is from the ophthalmic division of the trigeminal nerve, but the motor part is from the facial nerve.
  - Afferent defect (trigeminal nerve lesion): depression or absence of direct and consensual blinking reflex.
  - Efferent defect (facial nerve lesion): depression or absence of blinking reflex only on the side of facial weakness.
- **Jaw jerk reflex**: Ask patient to let his or her mouth fall open slightly. Put your index finger on the jaw and tap lightly with a tendon hammer. Normal response is slight closure of the mouth or no response. An exaggerated response implies an upper motor neuron (UMN) lesion (e.g. pseudobulbar palsy).

Facial nerve (VII)

- **Motor**: Ask the patient to frown and then raise his or her eyebrows, to close their eyes and stop you from opening them, to show you their teeth, to blow out their cheeks and purse their lips (all movements should be tested against resistance). Raising the eyebrows can differentiate between a UMN and a lower motor neuron (LMN) lesion (see Section 6.2).

- **Sensory**: Taste to anterior two-thirds of tongue.
- **Hyperacusis**: Ask the patient if noise sounds unpleasantly loud (facial nerve supplies stapedius; paralysis of the muscle prevents normal damping of sound).

Vestibulocochlear nerve (VIII)

- **Hearing:**
  - Whisper a number in the patient's ear whilst covering the other one. Ask the patient to repeat what he heard.
  - **Rinne's** and **Weber's** tests (see MICRO-facts, p. 16).
- **Vestibular**: Ask the patient if he or she has had any dizziness or problems with balance. Perform the Dix–Hallpike manoeuvre or other tests of vestibular function if appropriate.

Glossopharyngeal (IX) and vagus (X) nerves

- Ask the patient if he or she has had any problems swallowing. Ask the patient to say 'ah' and observe the movement of the palate and uvula. The uvula deviates towards the normal side in a vagal nerve palsy.
- Elicit the **gag reflex** by gently touching the back of the throat with a tongue depressor. Normal response is contraction of the soft palate.
- **Speech**: Listen to spontaneous speech and observe volume, clarity and rhythm.
  - Dysphonia may present with reduced speech volume, and the voice may sound husky.
  - Ask the patient to cough; a bovine quality indicates abnormal vocal cord function.
  - Test for dysarthria: ask to the patient to repeat phrases such as 'yellow lorry' (tongue [lingual] sounds) and 'baby hippopotamus' (lip [labial] sounds) and vocalise the vowel sounds.
  - Assess for dysphasia (receptive, expressive, conductive, etc.).

Accessory nerve (XI)

- **Sternocleidomastoid**: Ask the patient to turn his or her head towards their right shoulder whilst you provide resistance with your hand placed on the right side of the patient's chin. Repeat for the other side.
- **Trapezius**: Ask the patient to shrug shoulders whilst you provide counterforce.

Hypoglossal nerve (XII)

- Examine the patient's tongue at rest in the floor of mouth for fasciculation and wasting. Ask the patient to extend the tongue and observe for deviation towards the paralysed side. Ask the patient to push the tongue into his or her cheek on each side and test power by resistance.

Clinical neurology

LIMB EXAMINATION

Inspection

- Muscle wasting, scars, tremor, fasciculation and deformity.
- **Arm drift**: Ask patient to hold out both hands, palms facing upwards, arms extended and eyes closed. Note any pronator drift, due to:
  - **UMN lesion**: drift down and medial due to weakness. Forearm pronates, fingers may flex.
  - **Loss of proprioception**: drift in any direction.
  - **Cerebellar disease**: drift upwards due to hypotonia.

Tone

- Assessed by passive movement of the patient's limbs.
- Pyramidal (UMN) spasticity:
  - **Supinator catch**: On holding the patient's hand with the elbow flexed and quickly rotating the forearm, there is break in the smooth movement on supination.
  - **'Clasp-knife' effect**: On holding the patient's hand and extending the elbow, increased tone suddenly gives way to low tone.
- Extrapyramidal rigidity:
  - **'Lead pipe' rigidity**: increased tone throughout the movement of limb.
  - **'Cogwheel' rigidity**: caused by lead pipe rigidity combined with a tremor.

Power

- Assess power of all the major muscle groups.
- Weakness reported by the patient may be undetectable on examination. Functional tests (squatting, climbing stairs, etc.) may be useful.
- The pattern of any weakness should be categorised as this may suggest an underlying cause:
  - **Pyramidal** (weak upper limb extensors and lower limb flexors): upper motor neuron pathology (e.g. stroke, brain tumour, spinal cord disease).
  - **Proximal**: muscle or NMJ disease.
  - **Distal**: peripheral nerve.
- Muscle power is graded using the Medical Research Council (MRC) scale for muscle power:
  - **0**: no visible muscle contraction;
  - **1**: visible muscle contraction but no movement;
  - **2**: movement of limb with elimination of gravity (e.g. hip abduction);
  - **3**: movement against gravity but not against resistance from examiner;
  - **4**: movement against some resistance from examiner;
  - **5**: normal power against resistance.

Reflexes

- The following deep tendon reflexes should be elicited: biceps, triceps, supinator, knee and ankle.
- Babinski's sign ('upgoing plantars'): pressure on the sole of the foot should produce plantar flexion of the toes. In UMN lesions, scratching the sole produces reflex dorsiflexion (extension) due to the loss of normal inhibitory control.
- Responses are documented as:
  - hyperactive/'brisk' (+++);
  - normal (++);
  - diminished (+);
  - absent (–);
  - when only present using reinforcement (±).
- Ankle clonus:
  - rhythmic series of contractions caused by sudden passive dorsiflexion of the ankle;
  - briskly dorsiflex the foot whilst supporting the leg with the knee flexed and thigh externally rotated;
  - less than 5 beats of plantar flexion of the ankle is normal, but sustained clonus is a sign of an UMN lesion.

Coordination

- **Finger-nose test:**
  - Ask the patient to move a finger between his or her nose and your finger, ensuring a good amount of reach, repeating the action as quickly as possible.
  - In cerebellar or sensory ataxia, the patient may tend to fall short or overshoot your finger (past-pointing). In more severe disease, there may be tremor of the finger as it approaches the target finger or nose (intention tremor).
- **Rapid alternating movements:**
  - Hold one hand flat, palm up, and demonstrate the act of turning the other hand over repeatedly on it as quickly and regularly as possible. Ask the patient to copy your movements.
  - Dysdiadochokinesis is an inability to perform this action, a feature of cerebellar disease.
- **Heel-shin test:** Ask the patient to lift one leg and place the heel of that leg on the opposite knee. The heel should then be slid up and down the shin between the knee and ankle. It is abnormal if the heel moves away from the line of the shin.

Sensation

- Should be tested in all dermatomes. If a deficit is identified, the extent should be mapped out in more detail.

Clinical neurology

- **Soft touch** (dorsal columns): Use cotton wool, first demonstrating the normal sensation on the patient's sternum.
- **Pain/temperature sensation** (spinothalamic tract): Ask patient to say whether he or she feels a pin as sharp or blunt.
- **Proprioception** (dorsal columns): Hold the distal interphalangeal joint of the middle finger by the lateral aspects and demonstrate up-and-down movements to the patient. Then ask the patient to close the eyes and say whether movement is up or down as you move the joint randomly. If impaired, move to a more proximal joint.
- **Vibration** (dorsal columns): Ask the patient to close the eyes and place a 128-Hz tuning fork on the most distal bony prominence; ask the patient when the vibrations are detected and when the patient feels it stop (ensure the patient can differentiate between contact with the tuning fork and vibration). If impaired, move proximally.

Gait

- Ask the patient to walk normally, heel to toe, on the toes and on the heels (see the Gait abnormalities on page 17).
- **Romberg's test:**
  - Ask the patient to stand with feet together and then to close his or her eyes.
  - The test is positive if unsteadiness increases (due to loss of proprioception in sensory ataxia); this does not occur with cerebellar ataxia.

2.3 COMMON INVESTIGATIONS

NEUROPHYSIOLOGICAL INVESTIGATIONS

- **Electroencephalography (EEG):**
  - Multiple electrodes placed on the scalp measure the electrical activity of the brain.
  - Used (under expert supervision) to classify seizure type, assessment and localization for surgery, and in diagnosis of non-epileptic seizures (in conjunction with video telemetry).
  - Other indications include sleep disorders and suspected encephalitis.
- **Electromyography (EMG):**
  - Needle electrodes inserted into muscle examine the electrical activity produced.
  - Normal muscle at rest is electrically silent. In dennervated muscle at rest, spontaneous activity may be seen (e.g. positive sharp waves, fibrillation potentials and fasciculations).
  - Indications include myopathy and motor neuron disease.

- **Nerve conduction studies**:
  - Electrical stimuli are applied to nerves and muscles via a surface electrode.
  - A decrease in conduction velocity generally implies demyelination, whereas a reduction in amplitude suggests axonal loss.
  - Indications include peripheral neuropathies.

IMAGING

- **Computed tomography (CT)**:
  - **Advantages**: CT is faster, cheaper and often better than magnetic resonance imaging (MRI) for examining fresh blood and bony structures.
  - **Disadvantages**: Resolution is poorer than MRI, poor at imaging the posterior fossa and high radiation dose.
- **Magnetic resonance imaging**:
  - Diffusion-weighted imaging (DWI) detects areas where water diffusion has become restricted (e.g. stroke).
  - Magnetic resonance angiography (MRA) and venography (MRV) produce images of the cerebral and cervical blood vessels and are useful for investigating cerebral circulation stenosis or aneurysms.
  - **Advantages**: Absence of ionizing radiation (unlike CT/X-ray), highly detailed images and better resolution of structures surrounded by bone (e.g. spinal cord). Essential to detect demyelination and syrinx.
  - **Disadvantages**: Cannot be performed in patients with pacemakers as the magnetic field interferes with their function or in some patients with metallic foreign bodies (e.g. prostheses, surgical clips).
- **Catheter arteriography**:
  - A catheter passed via a large artery allows injection of a contrast agent into the cerebral arterial tree, which is imaged with a series of cranial radiographs.
  - Indications include imaging for detection of aneurysms and arteriovenous malformations and embolisation of aneurysms and vascular malformations.

LUMBAR PUNCTURE (CEREBROSPINAL FLUID ANALYSIS)

- **Indications**:
  - suspected meningitis/encephalitis;
  - subarachnoid haemorrhage;
  - investigation of other neurological conditions (e.g. multiple sclerosis or polyneuropathy).
- **Contraindications**:
  - raised intracranial pressure (unless proven communicating hydrocephalus);

Clinical neurology

- infection at the proposed puncture site;
- haemodynamic instability;
- coagulopathy;
- focal neurological deficit.
- **Complications**:
  - post-lumbar puncture low-pressure headache: headache that is worse when upright, occurs within 24 hours of the procedure and lasts 3–4 days;
  - infection, haemorrhage or, rarely, trauma to the nerve roots.

Part II

Neurological zones

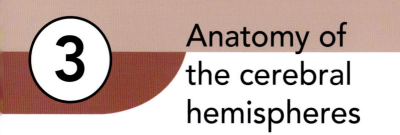

3 Anatomy of the cerebral hemispheres

3.1 ANATOMICAL DIAGRAMS (FIGS. 3.1 AND 3.2)

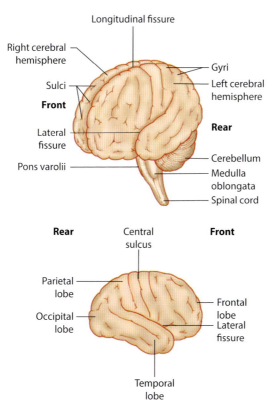

Fig. 3.1 Diagram of the brain, including frontal, parietal, temporal and occipital lobes with major sulci marked.

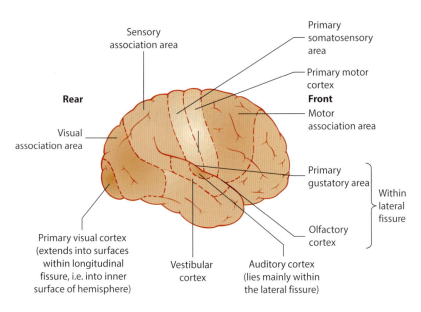

Fig. 3.2 Diagram of primary motor (frontal lobe) and primary sensory (parietal lobe) cortex separated by the central sulcus.

3.2 GROSS ANATOMY AND FUNCTION

- The cerebrum is divided into two hemispheres, which are subdivided into the four lobes: frontal, parietal, temporal and occipital.
- The cerebral cortex is the outermost layer of the cerebrum and is where higher cognitive processes take place (language, thought, memory etc.).
  - The cortex is folded into grooves or **sulci**; an area between grooves is a **gyrus**. Important functions may be localised to a single gyrus (see further discussion this chapter) or be more diffuse.
  - Many connections exist between cortical areas and deeper structures.
- Different cerebral functions may be attributed to the four lobes, and damage to an area (stroke, tumour) can produce a predictable deficit (significant variation occurs):
  - **Frontal lobe**: executive function (planning, social functioning, etc.); personality, emotional responses, some memory function. Contains motor areas.
  - **Parietal lobe**: integration of sensory input (contains somatosensory and visual areas).
  - **Temporal lobe**: memory (medial temporal lobe, hippocampus); auditory function.
  - **Occipital lobe**: visual processing.

3.3 PRIMARY MOTOR AND PRIMARY SENSORY CORTEX

- The primary motor cortex (M1) occupies the precentral gyrus (frontal lobe). The premotor cortex is anterior to this.
- The primary sensory cortex (S1) occupies the post-central gyrus (parietal lobe).
  - M1 and S1 are in the cerebral cortex but are notable for their **direct** contact with deep structures.
    - M1 contains motor neurons that extend directly to the ventral horn of the spinal cord to direct muscle movement.
    - S1 is the first cortical area to receive sensory input from the peripheral nervous system.
- M1 and S1 are connected to the thalamus and spinal cord via the **internal capsule** (see Chapter 4, Basal ganglia and subcortical structures).
- Both M1 and S1 contain a **topographic map** of the contralateral body, the '**homunculus**' (see **Fig. 3.3**):

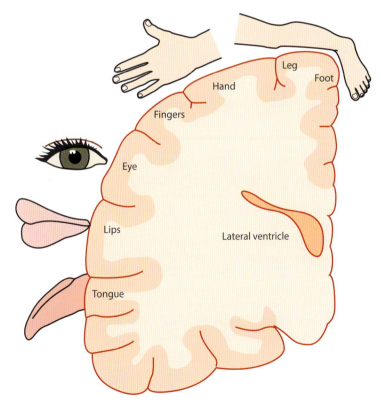

Fig. 3.3 Diagram showing representation of the body across S1.

- Inferior structures (e.g. lower limb) are located more medially, and superior structures (e.g. upper limb, face) are located more laterally.

MICRO-print

Spastic paraparesis is usually related to spinal cord injury. However, it may be due to cerebral cortex pathology, most commonly **cerebral palsy.**

- A rare cause is a **parasagittal meningioma** in the midline, as this will compress the primary motor cortex bilaterally (see **Fig. 3.4**).
- The topographic map across the primary motor cortex dictates that the legs are represented in the midline; therefore, the meningioma will produce a UMN pattern of weakness in both legs (a spastic paraparesis).

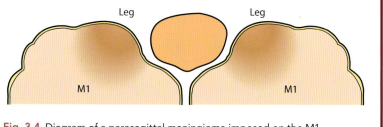

Fig. 3.4 Diagram of a parasagittal meningioma imposed on the M1 topographic map.

3.4 BROCA'S AREA AND WERNICKE'S AREA

- **Broca's area**: involved in the **production** of language and syntax. Located in the frontal lobe (posterior inferior frontal gyrus).
  - Damage to Broca's area in the dominant hemisphere produces **expressive dysphasia**, an inability to form words into comprehensible language.
    - Speech is non-fluent – laboured speech (telegrammatic) with few words, but meaning usually retained.
- **Wernicke's area**: involved in comprehension and meaning. Located in temporal lobe (posterior superior temporal gyrus).
  - Damage to Wernicke's area in the dominant hemisphere produces **receptive dysphasia** (i.e. an inability to comprehend the meaning of language).
    - The speech produced by such a patient may retain a normal rhythm and syntax (fluency) but be without meaning.

- Broca's and Wernicke's areas are joined by the arcuate fasciculus, lesions of which produce a conductive aphasia in which repetition is severely impaired.
- Global aphasia occurs due to damage to all the cortical speech centres. Comprehension is impaired, and speech output is limited to single words or noises.

MICRO-print

Testing of function of Broca's area and Wernicke's area should be part of a standard neurological examination. It can be done as follows:

- Ask the patient to follow a three-stage command described only by speech, such as, "Take this paper in your right hand, fold it in half and place it on the floor." Completion of this task successfully requires normal functioning of Wernicke's area.
- Ask the patient to correctly name commonly used objects, such as a pen and a watch. This requires both understanding and production of language (i.e. normal functioning of both Broca's area and Wernicke's area).

3.5 PRIMARY VISUAL CORTEX (V1)

- The primary visual cortex (V1) is located around the calcarine sulcus in each occipital lobe.
  - It is the first relay point for afferent visual information from the retina. Fibres project to other visual centres in the occipital lobe.
- The **contralateral visual field** is mapped across V1 in a given hemisphere.
- See **Figs. 3.5** and **3.6**.

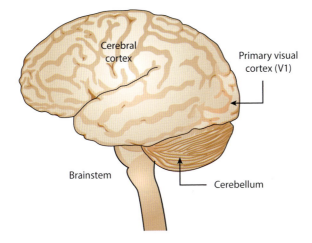

Fig. 3.5 Primary visual cortex (VI) is located at the occipital pole.

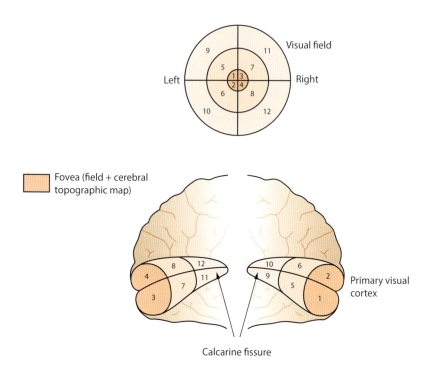

Fig. 3.6 Diagram of retinotopic map across VI.

MICRO-facts

- The occipital lobe is supplied by the posterior cerebral artery, although the occipital pole (the area of the occipital cortex that represents the macula area of the retina) receives a collateral blood supply from the middle cerebral artery (MCA).
- In a posterior artery stroke that would otherwise produce a complete homonymous hemianopia, the collateral supply to the occipital pole produces **macular sparing**, that is, sparing of the central portion of the visual field.

3.6 MENINGES

- The brain and spinal cord are covered by the three layers of the meninges (see **Fig. 3.7**).
- **Dura mater**: consists of two layers; the periosteal layer closely overlies the skull, and the meningeal layer lies deep to this.

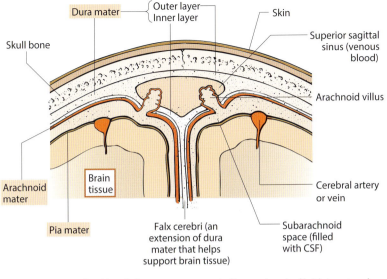

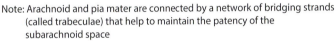

Note: Arachnoid and pia mater are connected by a network of bridging strands (called trabeculae) that help to maintain the patency of the subarachnoid space

Fig. 3.7 Diagram of the meninges layers in cross section, including skin, periosteum, bone, dura mater (periosteal and meningeal layer), epidural potential space, subdural potential space, arachnoid space, subarachnoid space filled with CSF, pia mater, brain. Also included are bridging veins.

- The dura forms several folds that dive down between intracranial structures:
  - The **falx cerebri** separates the cerebral hemispheres.
  - The **tentorium cerebelli** divides the occipital lobes and the cerebellum/brainstem.
  - The **falx cerebelli** lies in the posterior fossa and partially separates the cerebellar hemispheres.
- The space between the layers of dura mater contains the **venous sinuses**.
  - Veins that drain into the venous sinuses from deep structures cross the potential subdural space. These bridging veins are vulnerable to damage in trauma, which leads to a **subdural haematoma** (see Section 12.3).
- **Arachnoid mater**: lies deep to the dura but does not line the cerebral sulci.
  - Subarachnoid space: space between the arachnoid and pia mater that contains the cerebrospinal fluid (CSF).
  - Small protrusions through the dura into the sagittal venous sinus (**arachnoid granulations**) allow some drainage of CSF into the blood.

- **Pia mater**: closely adheres to the tissue of the brain.
- The meninges are one of the few pain-sensitive intracranial structures, and irritation will produce signs/symptoms of meningism (see Section 19.1).

MICRO-print

An **epidural haematoma** (see Section 12.2) may be caused by trauma to the thin part of the skull, the **pterion**. This overlies the **middle meningeal artery**, which is responsible for the majority of the blood supply to the meninges.

- Fracture of the pterion results in a tear of the middle meningeal artery and subsequent bleeding into the potential space between the dural layers.
- The bleed is **arterial**; therefore, the haematoma expands more acutely than a **venous** subdural haematoma.

3.7 VASCULAR ANATOMY OF THE BRAIN

THE ANTERIOR CIRCULATION

- The anterior circulation comprises the anterior and middle cerebral arteries, which stem from the internal carotid artery, and supplies most of the cerebral cortex, excluding the occipital lobe. See **Fig. 3.8** for anterior circulation, and **Fig. 3.9** for arterial territories.
  - The anterior circulation can be affected by all causes of stroke. The internal carotid artery is also vulnerable to dissection.

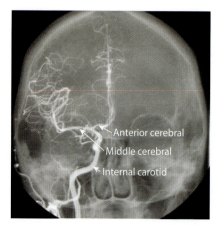

Fig. 3.8 Angiogram of the anterior circulation, including the internal and external carotids.

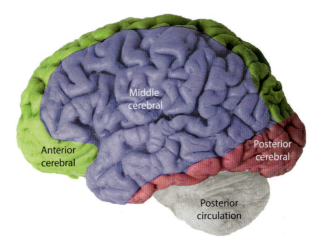

Fig. 3.9 Diagram of area supplied by the ACA, MCA and PCA.

- Middle cerebral artery (MCA):
    - Supplies almost the entire convex surface of the brain, including the lateral parietal, frontal and temporal lobes.
    - Occlusion of the MCA is responsible for 90% of ischaemic strokes.
- Anterior cerebral artery (ACA):
    - Supplies the medial surface of the parietal and frontal lobes.

THE POSTERIOR/VERTEBROBASILAR CIRCULATION (SEE FIG. 3.10)

- The vertebrobasilar/posterior circulation is derived from the basilar and vertebral arteries and supplies the occipital cortex, brainstem, cerebellum and anterior spinal cord.
    - The **posterior cerebral artery** is a branch of the basilar artery and supplies parts of the midbrain, subthalamic nucleus and occipital cortex (including primary visual cortex).

MICRO-print

There are a number of eponymous posterior circulation stroke syndromes:

- **Wallenberg syndrome** (lateral medullary syndrome): occlusion of the posterior inferior cerebellar artery (PICA) results in loss of pain and temperature sense, affecting the **ipsilateral face** and **contralateral body.** Also, ipsilateral Horner's syndrome, cerebellar signs, vertigo and palatal weakness.
- **Weber syndrome**: midbrain infarction as a result of occlusion of paramedian branches of the posterior cerebral artery resulting in ipsilateral III nerve palsy and contralateral hemiparesis.

Neurological zones

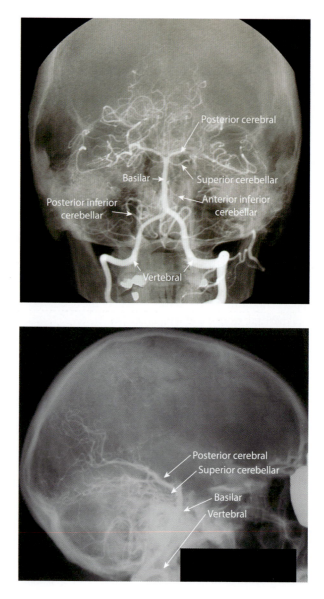

Fig. 3.10 Angiogram showing the posterior circulation including vertebral arteries, anterior spinal artery, basilar artery, posterior cerebral arteries and posterior inferior cerebellar arteries.

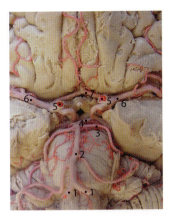

Fig. 3.11 Specimen demonstrating circle of Willis. 1: Left and right vertebral arteries; 2: Basilar artery; 3: Superior cerebellar artery; 4: Posterior cerebral artery; 5: Internal carotid artery; 6: Middle cerebral artery; 7: Anterior cerebral artery.

3.8 THE CIRCLE OF WILLIS (SEE FIG. 3.11)

- The circle of Willis represents the connection of the anterior and posterior circulation in a manner that allows redundancy: If one or more of the supplying arteries should be disrupted, the others can take over its end-arterial supply.
- Berry aneurysms are most often found in the circle of Willis and are a common cause of subarachnoid haemorrhage if they rupture.
  - A posterior communicating artery aneurysm commonly causes a palsy of the closely related III nerve (see Section 6.2).

3.9 VENOUS CIRCULATION AND VENOUS SINUSES (SEE FIG. 3.12)

- The venous sinuses are cavities of venous blood between the layers of the dura mater.
  - The sinuses receive venous blood from the internal and external veins of the brain and CSF from the subarachnoid space.
  - The interconnected system of sinuses ultimately drains into the internal jugular vein.
- The cavernous sinuses run in the cavities bordered by the temporal and sphenoid bones, and several important structures pass through them (see Section 6.1, MICRO-print; **Table 6.1**).

Neurological zones

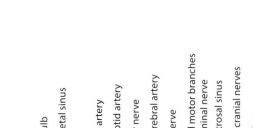

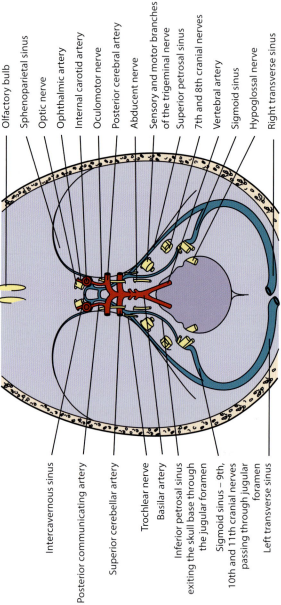

Olfactory bulb
Sphenoparietal sinus
Optic nerve
Ophthalmic artery
Internal carotid artery
Oculomotor nerve
Posterior cerebral artery
Abducent nerve
Sensory and motor branches of the trigeminal nerve
Superior petrosal sinus
7th and 8th cranial nerves
Vertebral artery
Sigmoid sinus
Hypoglossal nerve
Right transverse sinus

Intercavernous sinus
Posterior communicating artery
Superior cerebellar artery
Trochlear nerve
Basilar artery
Inferior petrosal sinus exiting the skull base through the jugular foramen
Sigmoid sinus – 9th, 10th and 11th cranial nerves passing through jugular foramen
Left transverse sinus

Fig. 3.12 Diagram of the system of venous sinuses and their relations.

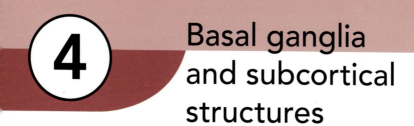

4 Basal ganglia and subcortical structures

4.1 ANATOMY OF THE SUBCORTICAL STRUCTURES

- The subcortical structures are connected to the cerebral cortex and include the basal ganglia, limbic system, internal capsule, thalamus, brainstem and cerebellum (see **Figs. 4.1** and **4.2**).

BASAL GANGLIA

- The basal ganglia are deep-brain structures that are highly involved in motor function:
    - motor learning and automation;
    - allow internally generated voluntary movements ('releasing') and suppress involuntary movements;
    - integrate emotion and other higher cerebral stimuli into movement.

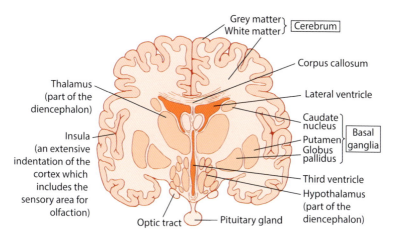

Fig. 4.1 Diagram of the brain in cross section showing the position of the various components of the basal ganglia.

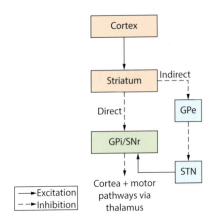

Fig. 4.2 Diagram of the direct and indirect pathways and their effect on basal ganglia inhibitory output to cortex and motor pathways. Loss of dopaminergic input from the substantia nigra pars compacta increases activity in the indirect pathway and reduces activity in the direct pathway. STN: subthalamic nucleus; GPe: external globus pallidus; GPi: internal blobus pallidus; SNr: substantia nigra pars reticulate.

- Composed of **claustrum, corpus striatum** and **substantia nigra**.
  - Corpus striatum is made up of **putamen, caudate nucleus** and **globus pallidus**.
    - **Caudate nucleus is** made up of head, body and tail. Separated from putamen by anterior limb of internal capsule.
    - **Putamen** is a mass of grey matter that is in close contact with the **globus pallidus** (together they form the lentiform nucleus). Separated from the thalamus by the posterior limb of the internal capsule.
- Described as part of the 'extra-pyramidal' motor system:
  - The motor pathways from the primary motor cortex to the descending corticospinal tracts are termed the *pyramidal tract*, as they decussate (intersect) at the medullary pyramids. The basal ganglia lie outside these tracts but are connected in a 'subcortical loop' (see MICRO-print 6.1).
  - Dopamine (released from the substantia nigra pars compacta) is an important neurotransmitter in the extra-pyramidal system, and imbalances are implicated in the pathogenesis of basal ganglia disorders (see below).

OTHER SUBCORTICAL STRUCTURES

- **Internal capsule**: white matter tracts that connect cortical areas (i.e., primary motor cortex, somatosensory cortex) to deeper structures (i.e., thalamus, brainstem) and carry fibres of the ascending and descending long tracts; made up of anterior and posterior limbs connected by the **genu**:
  - Anterior limb contains connections between thalamus and premotor cortex.

- Genu contains descending cortico-bulbar fibres traveling to cranial nerve nuclei.
- Posterior limb contains corticospinal fibres and ascending thalamocortical fibres from thalamus to sensory cortex.

> **MICRO-print**
> The internal capsule contains a very large number of ascending and descending fibres in a small area – even a very small infarction affecting this area may produce significant neurological deficit.

- **Thalamus**: mass of grey matter that forms the lateral wall of third ventricle. Function is as main sensory relay nucleus and to receive input from all main sensory modalities.
  - Contains lateral geniculate nucleus (visual tract) and medial geniculate nucleus (auditory tract).

4.2 PARKINSONIAN SYNDROMES

DEFINITION

- The Parkinsonian clinical syndromes are characterised by a combination of both negative and positive symptoms, including bradykinesia, resting tremor, muscular rigidity and postural instability.
- They are associated with an impairment of dopaminergic neurotransmission in the basal ganglia.

AETIOLOGY

- Parkinsonism is a feature of a number of different conditions:
  - idiopathic Parkinson's disease (IPD) (most common);
  - multiple system atrophy (MSA);
  - progressive supranuclear palsy (PSP);
  - corticobasal degeneration;
  - Lewy body dementia;
  - Wilson's disease;
  - toxic disorders (e.g., MPTP, methylphenyltetrahydropyridine);
  - drug-induced (dopamine antagonists) conditions;
  - cerebrovascular disease;
  - trauma (particularly repetitive head injury such as from boxing);
  - autoimmune encephalitis.

IDIOPATHIC PARKINSON'S DISEASE

DEFINITION

- A progressive neurodegenerative disorder of the dopaminergic neurons of the substantia nigra pars compacta.

PATHOPHYSIOLOGY

- Degeneration of the substantia nigra pars compacta impairs the dopaminergic input into the striatum.
- Cytoplasmic inclusions within neurons known as **Lewy bodies**, of which the major component is alpha-synuclein. Pathological changes are found throughout the basal ganglia and more widely in the cerebral cortex.

AETIOLOGY

- The mechanism of IPD is not well understood, but a number of risk factors have been associated with the disease:
  - **Genetics**: Genetic variants have been identified with mutations in genes, including *alpha-synuclein* and *parkin*; these genes appear to be associated with protein-processing pathways.
  - **MPTP**, as a contaminant of heroin, disrupts mitochondrial function and produces a rapid-onset parkinsonian syndrome.
  - **Environmental factors**:
    - Exogenous toxins and pesticides may increase the risk of developing the disease.
    - The risk of IPD is higher in those who live in a rural environment or close to industrial plants.
    - Smoking and caffeine consumption are inversely correlated with the risk of IPD.

EPIDEMIOLOGY

- **Prevalence**: ~120 people per 100,000 population.
- **Age**: Prevalence increases with age; mean age of onset is approximately 60 years old.
- **Gender**: It is more common in men (male-to-female ratio is approximately 1.5:1).

CLINICAL FEATURES

- Clinical features are asymmetrical in their onset.
- **Resting tremor**:
  - Coarse resting tremor (4–7 Hz) usually develops early in the disease.
  - Tremor typically starts in one arm, later becoming bilateral.
  - Often, 'pill rolling' occurs; the thumb moves rhythmically back and forwards on the palm of the hand.
  - It occurs at rest and improves with movement or sleep.
- **Bradykinesia**: slowness of initiating movement and progressive decrease in amplitude and rate of repetitive actions. Classical symptoms patients may report:
  - difficulty initiating movements such as walking or rising from a chair;
  - an expressionless face;

- monotonous, hypophonic (soft) speech;
- dysphagia;
- micrographia (decrease in the size of handwriting);
- slow and festinant (small shuffling steps whilst leaning forward, as if constantly falling forward) gait with reduced arm swing during walking.
- **Hypertonia**:
  - 'lead pipe' rigidity: uniform resistance to passive movement;
  - 'cog-wheel' rigidity: ratchety resistance to passive movement due to tremor superimposed on lead pipe rigidity.
- **Other features**:
  - Autonomic dysfunction producing urinary incontinence, postural hypotension and constipation.
  - Neuropsychiatric symptoms:
    - depression and dementia in up to 40% of patients;
    - psychotic symptoms, most often visual hallucinations.
  - Non-motor symptoms: may precede the motor symptoms and include loss of smell, constipation and REM (rapid eye movement) sleep disorders.

MICRO-print
If symptoms of dementia develop within the first 12 months of diagnosis of Parkinson's disease, it is termed **dementia with Lewy Bodies**. If it is diagnosed later, it is termed **Parkinson's disease dementia**.

INVESTIGATIONS

- Diagnosis is primarily clinical; trial of dopaminergic medication in suspected cases of IPD is often informative.
- SPECT (single-photon emission computed tomography) may be used when differentiation from essential tremor is difficult.

MANAGEMENT

- A **multidisciplinary team** (MDT) approach is used, including specialist neurologist, specialist nurses, an occupational therapist, a physiotherapist, a social worker and the general practitioner (GP).
- **Dopaminergic** therapy provides symptomatic improvement but has no effect on disease course or prognosis. It improves the negative symptoms of IPD but has less effect on tremor.
  - **Levodopa (L-dopa)**:
    - Dopamine-precursor that requires metabolism to dopamine by dopa-decarboxylase to become active.

- Given with a dopa-decarboxylase inhibitor that does not cross the blood-brain barrier (e.g. carbidopa) to minimize peripheral dopaminergic action and thus adverse effects.
- Long-term use at high dose can result in motor complications, including unpredictable mobility fluctuations (on-off phenomenon) and dyskinesia (see Section 1.2).

- **Dopamine agonists**:
  - These directly stimulate dopamine receptors.
  - Ropinirole or pramipexole is used as monotherapy in younger patients.
  - Apomorphine is given as a subcutaneous injection or continuous infusion to patients in the end stage of disease when other agents fail to control symptoms.
  - They can cause a psychotic reaction and increased risk-taking behaviour.
- **COMT (catechol-O-methyltransferase) inhibitors**:
  - These inhibit breakdown of dopamine by COMT and increase central dopamine availability.
  - COMT inhibitors are not suitable for use as a monotherapy but may be used as an adjunct to L-dopa.
- **Monoamine oxidase B (MAO-B) inhibitors**:
  - These inhibit the breakdown of dopamine in the central nervous system (CNS), thereby increasing nigrostriatal dopamine levels.
  - Examples include rasagiline and selegiline (note: multiple drug interactions).
- **Surgery**: Bilateral subthalamic nucleus or globus pallidus interna stimulation ('deep-brain stimulation') is useful in patients with intolerable side effects from medication.
- Non-motor symptoms of IPD require careful identification and management:
  - Psychotic symptoms:
    - may occur as a drug side effect or as a result of disease;
    - managed with atypical antipsychotics such as quetiapine;
  - Autonomic disturbances:
    - oxybutynin for overactive bladder;
    - oral amitriptyline or botulinum toxin injections into the salivary glands for sialorrhoea.

Prognosis

- There is no treatment available currently to slow the progression of IPD. Life expectancy is approximately 15 years from diagnosis.
- Aspiration pneumonia as a result of dysphagia is a common cause of mortality.
- Prognosis is better in patients with tremor-predominant disease as opposed to bradykinesia-dominant disease.

MULTIPLE SYSTEM ATROPHY (MSA)

- Progressive neurodegenerative disorder with an unknown aetiology affecting multiple sites in the CNS.
- Incidence is around 3 per 100,000 annually in the population aged over 50 years; mean age at onset is between 50 and 70 years.
- Pathogenesis is not fully understood; it is characterized by widespread **glial cytoplasmic inclusions** containing α-**synuclein** with associated neuronal loss in the basal ganglia, cerebellum, pons, inferior olivary nuclei and spinal cord.
- **Clinical features**:
    - parkinsonian symptoms with poor response to levodopa;
    - autonomic dysfunction – postural hypotension or urinary incontinence;
    - cerebellar symptoms;
    - corticospinal tract signs – 'upper motor neuron' pattern of weakness;
    - cognitive impairment in approximately 20%.
- Diagnosis is predominantly clinical; SPECT scanning will **not** distinguish IPD from MSA.
- Management of MSA is aimed at symptom control as there is no available therapy to reverse or slow disease progression.
- Median survival is 9 years from onset of symptoms.
- Poor prognostic factors include older age at onset, female gender and early autonomic failure.

PROGRESSIVE SUPRANUCLEAR PALSY

- A progressive neurodegenerative disorder of unknown aetiology, characterized by parkinsonism in combination with pseudobulbar palsy and dysfunction of eye movements and cognition.
- **Pathophysiology**: accumulation of neurofibrillary tangles containing phosphorylated tau protein in the basal ganglia, in the brainstem (including nuclei controlling eye movements and swallowing) and in the cerebral hemispheres, particularly the frontal cortex.
- Prevalence is approximately 6 per 100,000; incidence is equal in males and females.
- **Clinical features**: The onset of PSP is often relatively insidious and non-specific:
    - parkinsonian symptoms;
    - pseudobulbar palsy;
    - supranuclear ophthalmoplegia: Vertical eye movements are impaired first, followed by horizontal eye movements late in the disease course;
    - cognitive impairment in over 50% of cases, typically frontal in type.
- Diagnosis is clinical.

Neurological zones

- There is no effective treatment for PSP.
  - PSP-related parkinsonism is poorly responsive to dopaminergic therapy.
  - Symptoms such as sialorrhea may be managed as for IPD.
- Clinical course is variable, with mortality usually occurring 6–10 years after the onset of symptoms; infections and pulmonary complications are the main causes of death.

MICRO-print

Corticobasal degeneration

- There is significant cross over between PSP and corticobasal degeneration (CBD). CBD is also a **tau-opathy** that presents with parkinsonism and cognitive decline.
- CBD and PSP can often only be distinguished based on post-mortem neuropathological changes.
- Like PSP, there is no specific treatment for CBD, and the parkinsonian symptoms are often poorly responsive to dopaminergic agents.

WILSON'S DISEASE

DEFINITION

- An inherited defect of copper metabolism.

EPIDEMIOLOGY

- **Prevalence**: approximately 1 per 30,000 population.
- **Gender**: equally common in males and females.

AETIOLOGY

- Due to a mutation of a gene on chromosome 13 that codes for copper transporting ATPase (adenosine triphosphatase) with an autosomal recessive inheritance pattern.

PATHOPHYSIOLOGY

- The function of **copper-transporting ATPase** is disturbed such that copper incorporation into caeruloplasmin in the liver and its excretion into bile are impaired.
- Copper **accumulates in the liver**, causing oxidative damage
- The liver releases free copper into the bloodstream, which precipitates in other organs, particularly the **basal ganglia, kidneys** and **eyes**.

MICRO-facts

Kayser–Fleischer rings are the result of copper deposits in Descemet's membrane of the eye, resulting in a brownish-yellow ring in the outer rim of the cornea. They may be visible to the naked eye or by ophthalmoscopy, but usually slit-lamp examination is required. Kayser–Fleischer rings are **diagnostic** of Wilson's disease.

CLINICAL FEATURES (TABLE 4.1)

- Children usually present with liver disease; young adults may present with neuropsychiatric features.

Table 4.1 Clinical features of Wilson's disease

SYSTEM	CLINICAL FEATURES
Hepatic	Chronic hepatitis, progressing to cirrhosis Fulminant liver failure (±haemolytic anaemia)
Neurological	Asymmetrical tremor Parkinsonism Pseudobulbar palsy Dysarthria Dyskinesias Dystonias Dementia Gait disturbances Insomnia Seizures Migraine headaches
Psychiatric	Depression Psychoses Personality changes Neuroses
Ophthalmic	Kayser–Fleischer rings Sunflower cataracts (visible only on slit-lamp examination; do not cause visual loss)
Other	Blue nails Polyarthritis Hypermobile joints Grey skin Hypoparathyroidism

Neurological zones

INVESTIGATIONS

- Blood investigations show low **caeruloplasmin** levels and raised **unbound or 'free' copper.**
- The 24-hour urinary copper excretion is elevated (>100 μg/24 hours, normal < 40 μg/24 hours).
- **Liver biopsy**: Hepatic copper content is elevated.
- **MRI (magnetic resonance imaging) brain**: High signal in basal ganglia indicates copper deposition or basal ganglia degeneration or frontotemporal, cerebellar and brainstem atrophy.
- Molecular genetic testing confirms diagnosis.

MANAGEMENT

- **Pharmacological**:
  - **Copper chelators** (e.g. penicillamine) bind to and increase excretion of copper.
    - Levels of caeruloplasmin and blood and urinary copper should be monitored.
  - **Zinc** is used when copper levels have returned to normal.
    - It stimulates binding of copper by gut epithelium, preventing its absorption and transport to the liver.
- Liver transplantation may be necessary in severe hepatic disease.
- Family screening: First-degree relatives of asymptomatic homozygotes will require preventive treatment.

PROGNOSIS

- Lifelong treatment is required; without it, fatal liver failure occurs before the age of 40 years.
- Life expectancy is normal with treatment.

4.3 HUNTINGTON'S DISEASE

DEFINITION

- An inherited autosomal dominant, progressive neurodegenerative disorder associated with behavioural changes, chorea, dystonia and cognitive decline.

EPIDEMIOLOGY

- **Prevalence**: 5–7 per 100,000.
- **Age**: Onset is usually during middle age (mean age 35–44 years), but it may develop at any age.

AETIOLOGY

- It is an autosomal dominant inherited disorder.

- It is associated with expanded trinucleotide repeat (CAG) in a gene called *huntingtin* located on chromosome 4.
- Subsequent generations have more repeats and develop disease earlier than previous generations, a phenomenon known as anticipation.

PATHOPHYSIOLOGY

- The function of the *huntingtin* protein is not completely understood.
- Research suggests that expansions of *huntingtin* cause a toxic gain of function in the protein product.
- Neuropathological changes include cell loss and atrophy in the basal ganglia and cerebral cortex.

CLINICAL FEATURES

- Typically, there is a **prediagnostic phase** of up to 10 years with subtle changes in personality, cognition and motor control.
- **Symptomatic phase**:
  - Basal ganglia dysfunction: parkinsonism and positive symptoms such as chorea, hemiballismus and dystonia;
  - Cognitive dysfunction: impairment of executive function;
  - Neuropsychiatric symptoms: blunted affect, apathy, compulsive behaviour and mood disorder.

INVESTIGATIONS

- **Imaging**:
  - **MRI brain**: shows loss of striatal volume and enlargement of the frontal horns of the lateral ventricles in moderate-to-severe disease;
  - **PET** (positron emission tomographic) **scan**: shows a loss of function in the caudate nuclei.
- **Genetic testing** with demonstration of the repeat sequence is diagnostic.

MANAGEMENT

- There is currently no disease-modifying therapy; therefore, management is directed at symptom control only.
  - **Antidopaminergic** drugs are aimed at ameliorating the **positive** symptoms, including chorea.
  - **Dopaminergic drugs** may improve the parkinsonian symptoms.
  - **Antidepressants** and **antipsychotics** may be used for the neuropsychiatric symptoms.
- Genetic counselling should be offered to patients and family; there is a 50% chance of a patient's offspring being affected.

PROGNOSIS

- HD is progressive and death usually occurs within 15 years of diagnosis.

Neurological zones

MICRO-case

Idiopathic Parkinson's disease

A 65-year-old man presents to his GP with shaking in his right hand, reduced arm swing and difficulty walking. He feels like his arm is not working properly. He has noticed these changes gradually over the last 6 months. The patient's wife comments that his handwriting has recently changed, becoming much smaller.

Clinical examination shows a pill-rolling tremor, which is most pronounced at rest and reduces on movement. He has cogwheel rigidity in his right arm, an expressionless face and bradykinesia. The GP suspects Parkinson's disease and refers him to a neurologist.

Idiopathic Parkinson's disease is diagnosed, and the patient is initially started on ropinirole, a dopamine agonist. His case is discussed in the MDT meeting, and he is assigned a specialist nurse. He is also referred for physiotherapy and occupational therapy.

The patient was reviewed regularly by the MDT, and his symptoms were monitored and treated appropriately.

Summary points

- Symptoms often start unilaterally and then spread to both sides.
- Tremor is usually one of first signs and is classically pill rolling.
- L-Dopa is the most effective treatment for Parkinson's, but its efficacy reduces with time, and the on-off phenomenon may occur. Patients are therefore often started on a dopamine agonist.
- Regular multidisciplinary reviews are essential.

5 Cerebrospinal fluid and ventricular system

5.1 CEREBROSPINAL FLUID AND ANATOMY OF THE VENTRICLES (SEE FIG. 5.1)

- The central nervous system (CNS) effectively floats in cerebrospinal fluid (CSF), which provides it with mechanical and immunological protection.
- CSF is produced in the choroid plexus (in the lateral ventricles) from blood.
  - It then flows from the lateral ventricles into the third ventricle and then into the fourth ventricle via the cerebral aqueduct.
  - Passage of CSF from the fourth ventricle into the subarachnoid space is via the median aperture (foramen of Magendie) and lateral apertures (foramina of Lushka); pooling occurs in cisterns before circulating around the spinal cord and onto the lumbar cistern.
- CSF is reabsorbed into the venous system from the subarachnoid space via the arachnoid villi, which are projections of the arachnoid into the dural sinuses.
- The central canal of the spinal cord connects with the lumbar cistern at L3–5, which is the site of CSF sampling during a lumbar puncture procedure.
- CSF is also reabsorbed via the spinal nerve root pockets into the lymphatic system.

5.2 HYDROCEPHALUS

Definition

- **Hydrocephalus**
  - An increase in cerebrospinal fluid (CSF) volume within the cerebral ventricles.
  - Results in a pathological increase in pressure on the surrounding structures and eventually raised intracranial pressure (ICP).
  - Usually due to impaired reabsorption or obstruction of CSF flow; rarely occurs due to overproduction of CSF.

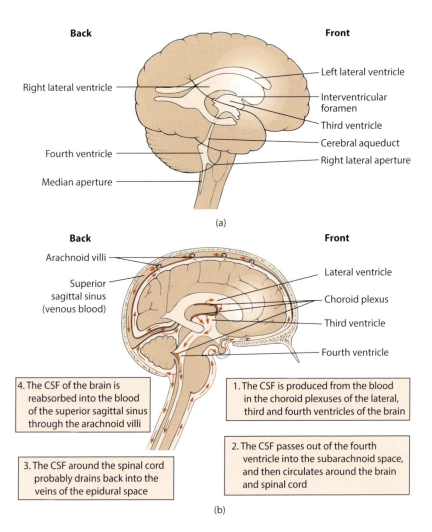

Fig. 5.1 (a) Diagram of the lateral ventricles, third and fourth ventricles and cerebral aqueduct. (b) Diagram showing the location CSF production, circulation and reabsorption.

- **Non-communicating or obstructive hydrocephalus**
  - Obstruction of CSF flow along one or more of the passages within the ventricles or between the ventricles and subarachnoid space.
  - CSF volume accumulates behind the obstruction.
- **Communicating hydrocephalus**
  - An increase in CSF volume due to the blockage of CSF after it exits the ventricles. CSF may still flow between ventricles.

Neurological zones

MICRO-facts

Lumbar puncture in hydrocephalus

A **lumbar puncture** is potentially dangerous in obstructive hydrocephalus as it may precipitate cerebellar herniation:

- Reduction in volume within the lumbar cistern generates negative pressure, which pulls the cerebellar tonsils downwards through the foramen magnum (also known as coning). This may lead to coma and death.

In communicating hydrocephalus, however, a lumbar puncture may therapeutically reduce the CSF pressure.

MICRO-print

Ex vacuo hydrocephalus

Expansion of the ventricular system secondary to shrinkage of adjacent brain tissue (e.g. by atrophy). There is no increase in CSF pressure and no symptoms of hydrocephalus.

MICRO-print

Normal-pressure hydrocephalus

- A syndrome of chronic hydrocephalus in the absence of a measurable raise in CSF pressure. It may follow head injury, meningitis or subarachnoid haemorrhage; however the cause is often idiopathic.
- There is a triad of **dementia, gait disturbance** and **incontinence**.
- Brain imaging shows ventricular enlargement without reciprocal effacement of sulci.
- It should be investigated with a timed walk, before and after the removal of 50 mls of CSF fluid by lumbar puncture.
- If there is a marked improvement in gait, the insertion of a ventriculoperitoneal (VP) shunt may be considered appropriate management.

EPIDEMIOLOGY

- **Incidence of congenital hydrocephalus**: 0.4 to 3.16 per 1000 live births.
- Incidence of acquired hydrocephalus is unknown; approximately 100,000 patients have shunts fitted every year in the developed world.

Neurological zones

Aetiology

- A third of cases of acquired hydrocephalus are **idiopathic**; this includes idiopathic intracranial hypertension, which is a communicating hydrocephalus.
- **Risk factors** for congenital hydrocephalus:
  - pre-eclampsia;
  - alcohol use during pregnancy;
  - lack of antenatal care.
- See **Table 5.1**

Table 5.1 Causes of hydrocephalus

	OBSTRUCTIVE	COMMUNICATING
Acquired	• **Acquired aqueduct stenosis** (adhesions following infections or haemorrhage) • **Supratentorial masses** causing tentorial herniation, intraventricular haematoma • **Tumours** – ventricular (e.g. colloid cyst, pineal tumours, tumours of posterior fossa) • **Abscesses/granuloma** • **Arachnoid cysts**	• **Thickening of leptomeninges** or involvement of arachnoid granulations (e.g. infection, subarachnoid haemorrhage, carcinomatous meningitis) • **Increased CSF viscosity** (e.g. high protein content) • **Excessive CSF production** (e.g. choroid plexus papilloma [rare])
Congenital	• **Aqueduct stenosis** • **Dandy Walker syndrome** (atresia of the foramen of Magendie and Luschka) • **Chiari malformation** • **Vein of Galen aneurysm**	

Clinical features

Presentation in young children prior to the fusing of the fontanelles is different from that in older children and adults.

- Infants and young children
  - Acute-onset hydrocephalus:
    - irritability;
    - impaired consciousness level;
    - vomiting.

- Gradual-onset hydrocephalus:
  - mental retardation;
  - failure to thrive.
- Regardless of the rate of onset:
  - tense anterior fontanelle;
  - increased head circumference.
- Adults
  - Acute-onset hydrocephalus:
    - impaired upwards gaze; due to pressure transmission to midbrain tectum;
    - signs and symptoms of raised ICP.
  - Gradual-onset hydrocephalus:
    - dementia;
    - gait ataxia;
    - incontinence.

INVESTIGATIONS

- **Imaging:**
  - **Skull X-ray**: Enlarged skull and erosion of the posterior clinoids may be seen, suggesting chronically raised pressure.
  - **CT brain**: Ventricular enlargement will be visible; different patterns can help differentiate communicating hydrocephalus and obstructive hydrocephalus.
  - **MRI brain**: Ventricular expansion is present; neoplasms or periventricular lucency may be seen.
  - **Cranial ultrasound**: Used to detect ventricular enlargement in infants (only possible prior to closure of fontanelles).
- Intracranial pressure (ICP) monitoring.

MANAGEMENT

- Treat the underlying cause.
- Diuretics may provide some relief before definitive intervention.
- **Surgical intervention**:
  - Acute hydrocephalus:
    - ventriculostomy (surgical opening of the ventricle) or shunt placement and CSF drainage;
    - drainage of CSF via repeat lumbar punctures or insertion of a lumbar drain in cases of communicating hydrocephalus;
  - Gradual-onset hydrocephalus:
    - insertion of a VP or ventriculoatrial (VA) shunt.

Neurological zones

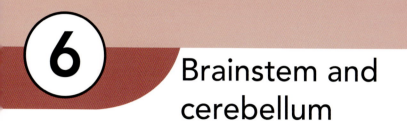

6 Brainstem and cerebellum

6.1 ANATOMY OF BRAINSTEM AND CEREBELLUM (SEE FIG. 6.1)

BRAINSTEM

- Made up of **midbrain, pons** and **medulla**.
- **Midbrain**:
  - Connects diencepahalon (thalamus and hypothalamus) to pons and medulla;
  - Dorsal surface forms the four colliculi:
    - two superior colliculi that are part of visual control system and mediate smooth pursuit and saccades;
    - two inferior colliculi that are involved in the auditory system.
  - Midbrain also contains red nucleus, fibres of the substantia nigra, the pretectal nucleus and the Edinger–Westphal nucleus, and the oculomotor nerve nucleus.
- **Pons**: connects midbrain and medulla and contains several nuclei (including several cranial nerve nuclei), as well as descending and ascending tracts.
- **Medulla**:
  - Superior relation is the pons and becomes continuous with the spinal cord posteriorly through the foramen magnum.
  - Anterior surface has anteromedian fissure that forms two swellings, the **medullary pyramids** (descending corticospinal tracts decussate here).
  - Fourth ventricle lies posteriorly between medulla and cerebellum.
- The medulla contains the nuclei that are vital for basic functions, such as the respiratory centre.

MICRO-print

Subcortical loops

The basal ganglia and cerebellum do not lie directly in the main motor and sensory pathways between the cerebral cortex and sensory organs or muscles. However, they are connected to both motor and sensory

continued...

continued...

areas and do play an important role in **coordination of movement**. The cerebellum is thought to function as a calibrator of movement based on past sensory information, that is, **externally guided movement** (movements in reaction to external stimuli); this is reflected in **past-pointing** and **ataxia**, which occur when the cerebellum is damaged.

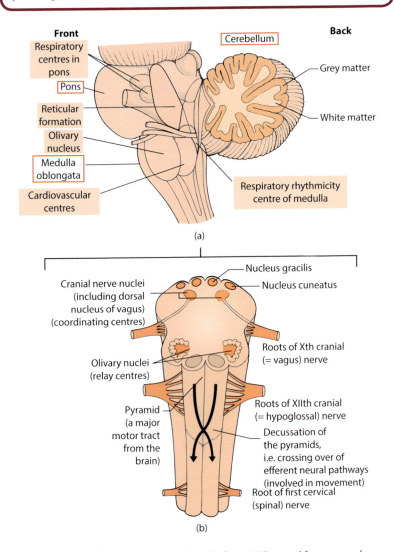

(a)

(b)

Fig. 6.1 Diagrams of the brainstem and cerebellum. (a) External features and position of the cardiovascular centres and respiratory centres; (b) Section through medulla oblongata.

CEREBELLUM

- The cerebellum lies in the posterior fossa.
- It is made up of two lateral **hemispheres** and a central **vermis**. The surface of the cerebellum is thrown into folds that mark out lobes – ventral portion of the hemispheres from flocculonodular lobes, which are separated from the rest of the cerebellum.
- Connections with the midbrain, pons and medulla are formed by the superior, middle and inferior cerebellar peduncles, respectively.
- The cerebellar cortex contains projections of afferent fibres, and white matter contains nuclei (largest is the dentate nucleus).
- The cerebellum receives inputs from ascending sensory pathways and vestibular and visual systems and has connections with the cerebral cortex and the basal ganglia. It functions to coordinate muscular actions and balance as well as muscular tone.
- **Blood supply**:
  - **Posterior inferior cerebellar artery**: branch of the vertebral artery that supplies posterior aspect of vermis and hemispheres.
  - **Anterior inferior cerebellar artery**: branch of the basilar artery that supplies anterolateral part of undersurface.
  - **Superior cerebellar artery**: branch of basilar artery that supplies superior aspect.

CRANIAL NERVES (SEE **FIG. 6.2**)

- These nerves are part of the peripheral nervous system (except the optic nerve, which is a central nervous system [CNS] structure).
- Connect the CNS to the sensory organs and muscles of the head and neck.
- Notably, the vagus nerve carries the parasympathetic supply to the majority of the thorax and abdomen.

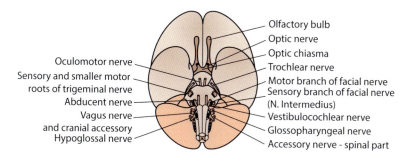

Olfactory bulb
Optic nerve
Optic chiasma
Oculomotor nerve
Trochlear nerve
Sensory and smaller motor
roots of trigeminal nerve
Motor branch of facial nerve
Sensory branch of facial nerve
Abducent nerve
(N. Intermedius)
Vagus nerve
Vestibulocochlear nerve
and cranial accessory
Glossopharyngeal nerve
Hypoglossal nerve
Accessory nerve - spinal part

Fig. 6.2 Diagram of origins of cranial nerves from the brainstem.

Neurological zones

MICRO-print

Anatomical relations of cranial nerve courses

- The VI cranial nerve, by nature of its long course, is vulnerable to raised intracranial pressure (ICP) and thus can be a **false localising sign**.
- Many of the cranial nerves are vulnerable to pathology at the **base of the skull** because of their course between the brainstem and their end-organ targets.
  - **Basal meningitis**: particularly affects cranial nerves III, IV, VI and VII.
- Cranial nerves II, III, IV, VI and V (ophthalmic branch) pass together though the **cavernous sinus** and thus form a specific pattern of deficit in cavernous sinus pathology, such as thrombosis. The same nerves subsequently pass through the **superior orbital fissure** and are thus vulnerable to orbital trauma, particularly if a 'blowout' fracture occurs.
- The anatomical course of the **VII nerve** is very important in many of the common causes of a palsy:
  - **Ramsay Hunt Syndrome**: In this syndrome, there is an association of a VII nerve palsy with a 'shingles' infection affecting the head and neck; most commonly, the mechanism is zoster infection affecting the geniculate ganglion within the temporal bone.
  - **Parotitis or parotid neoplasm**: VII nerve passes through the **parotid gland**; therefore, a palsy is not uncommon in these conditions.
- Cranial nerves IX, X and XI all pass through the **jugular foramen** and are thus vulnerable to its obstruction (e.g. by a glomus jugulare tumour or base-of-skull fracture).
- A lesion in the **cerebellopontine angle** such as an acoustic neuroma affects a number of cranial nerves as they leave the brainstem. Most commonly affected are cranial nerves VIII, V and VII.
- See **Table 6.1**.

Table 6.1 Cranial nerves

NAME	NUCLEI	COURSE	MOTOR FUNCTION	SENSORY FUNCTION	AUTONOMIC FUNCTION
Olfactory (I)	Anterior olfactory nucleus	Cribriform plate	None	Sense of smell	None
Optic (II)	Ganglion cells of retina	Optic canal	None	Vision	None
Oculomotor (III)	Oculomotor nucleus, Edinger-Westphal nucleus	Cavernous sinus, superior orbital fissure	Extraocular muscles except superior oblique and lateral rectus	None	Pupillary sphincter
Trochlear (IV)	Trochlear nucleus		Superior oblique muscle (SO4)	None	None
Abducens (VI)	Abducens nucleus		Lateral rectus muscle (LR6)	None	None
Trigeminal (V)	Trigeminal nucleus	Cavernous sinus (ophthalmic/maxillary divisions), superior orbital fissure (maxillary division)	Muscles of mastication	Sensation from skin of face	

(Continued)

Neurological zones

Table 6.1 (Continued)

NAME	NUCLEI	COURSE	MOTOR FUNCTION	SENSORY FUNCTION	AUTONOMIC FUNCTION
Facial (VII)	Facial nucleus, solitary nucleus, superior salivary nucleus	Internal acoustic canal, through parotid	Muscles of facial expression	Taste to anterior 2/3 of tongue	Secretomotor innervation to salivary glands (except parotid) and lacrimal gland
Vestibulocochlear (VIII)	Vestibular nuclei, cochlear nuclei	Internal acoustic canal	None	Hearing, rotation and gravity	None
Glossopharyngeal (IX)	Nucleus ambiguus, inferior salivary nucleus, solitary nucleus	Jugular foramen	Stylopharyngeus	Taste to posterior 1/3 of tongue	Secretomotor innervations to parotid gland
Vagus (X)	Dorsal vagal nucleus, nucleus ambiguus, solitary nucleus		Most muscles of larynx and pharynx	Taste to epiglottis	Parasympathetic supply to most thoracic and abdominal viscera above splenic flexure
Accessory (XI)	Nucleus ambiguus, spinal accessory nucleus		Sternocleidomastoid and trapezius	None	None
Hypoglossal (XII)	Hypoglossal nucleus	Hypoglossal canal	Muscles of tongue	None	None

6.2 CRANIAL NERVE PALSIES

OLFACTORY NERVE (I)

AETIOLOGY

- **Infective**: upper respiratory tract infection (usually transient).
- **Nasal pathology**: nasal polyps, enlarged turbinates.
- **Trauma**:
  - fracture of the cribiform plate;
  - vulnerable in pituitary surgery.
- **Malignancy**:
  - ethmoid sinus tumours;
  - meningioma of the olfactory groove.
- **Congenital**: Kallman's syndrome.

CLINICAL FEATURES

- Reduced or altered taste.
- Reduced or altered smell:
- Ammonia is **not** a useful olfactory stimulus as it activates pain fibres carried by the trigeminal nerve rather than olfactory fibres.

OPTIC NERVE (II)

- See Section 8.3.

OCULOMOTOR (III), TROCHLEAR (IV) AND ABDUCENS (VI) NERVES

- The III, IV and VI cranial nerves together supply the ocular muscles. They may be affected by disease processes singly or together.
- Notably, they travel together in the cavernous sinus and through the superior orbital fissure into the orbit (see previous MICRO-print on cranial nerve courses).
- As with the other cranial nerves, medullary disease may affect the nerve nuclei or intramedullary fibres. However, extramedullary lesions are more common.

Oculomotor (III) nerve

AETIOLOGY

- **Vascular**: most common cause in elderly.
  - Infarction: usually microvascular disease affecting extramedullary portion of nerve (e.g. diabetes); occasionally brainstem infarction affecting nucleus.
  - Compression by posterior communicating artery aneurysm.
  - Cavernous sinus disease: thrombosis, internal carotid artery aneurysm.
- **Inflammatory**:
  - sarcoidosis;
  - Miller Fisher syndrome;

- Tolosa–Hunt syndrome (granulomatous angiitis);
- basal meningitis.
- **Malignancy**:
  - skull base carcinoma;
  - compression by tumour at superior orbital fissure.
- **Trauma**: fractured base of the skull or the superior orbital fissure.

CLINICAL FEATURES

- At rest, the affected eye will be deviated **down** and **out**; diplopia occurs in all directions of gaze.
- Pupil dilation occurs due to loss of the parasympathetic supply to the pupillary sphincter.
- Ptosis.

MICRO-facts

Surgical versus medical III nerve palsy

- The parasympathetic fibres lie on the outer surface of the occulomotor nerve. Therefore, compressive causes (tumour, aneurysm) will cause pupillary dilation early in the disease course (**surgical palsy**).
- If the pupillary reflex is spared, this suggests a non-compressive cause of III nerve palsy (**medical palsy**); if this is an isolated neurological deficit, then the most common cause is microvascular infarction due to diabetes mellitus.

Trochlear (IV) nerve

AETIOLOGY

- Similar to oculomotor motor nerve palsy (not posterior communicating artery aneurysm).

CLINICAL FEATURES

- **Diplopia**:
  - Maximal on looking down and inwards.
  - Patients often report diplopia when walking down stairs or reading.
  - Patients may tilt their head to the affected side to compensate.

Abducens (VI) nerve

AETIOLOGY

- Similar to oculomotor nerve palsy (not posterior communicating artery aneurysm).
- Any pathology that increases ICP may lead to displacement of the brainstem, causing traction on the abducens nerves and uni- or bilateral palsies.

- Compression may also occur along its long intracranial course (see previous MICRO-print on cranial nerve courses).

CLINICAL FEATURES

- Inability to abduct the eye due to palsy of the lateral rectus muscle.
- Diplopia on lateral gaze towards the affected side.

TRIGEMINAL NERVE (V)

- The trigeminal nerve has three main branches: ophthalmic, maxillary and mandibular (see **Fig. 6.3**).
- Due to differences in their anatomical courses, disease processes may affect them all or singly.

AETIOLOGY

- **Inflammatory/infective**:
  - Herpes zoster infection:
    - Ophthalmic branch involvement may lead to residual corneal scarring (involvement of the tip of the nose, supplied by the nasociliary nerve, may precede corneal damage).
    - Persistent pain may occur in the affected area (post-herpetic neuralgia).
- **Neoplastic**: tumours of the cerebellopontine angle (e.g. acoustic neuroma).
- **Vascular**:
  - microvascular infarction;
  - compression in a cavernous sinus thrombosis (ophthalmic and maxillary divisions).
- **Trauma**: fracture of the superior orbital fissure.

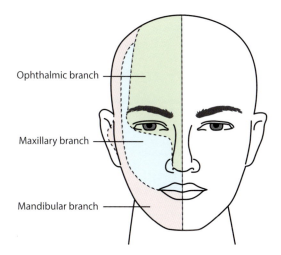

Ophthalmic branch

Maxillary branch

Mandibular branch

Fig. 6.3 Diagram showing the skin supplied by the three branches of the trigeminal nerve.

Neurological zones

CLINICAL FEATURES

- Absent corneal reflex (often first sign).
- Weakness of the muscles of mastication; in a unilateral lesion, the jaw may deviate to the affected side.
- Loss of facial sensation: Sensory loss involving all three divisions is suggestive of a lesion at the ganglion or sensory root (e.g. a cerebellopontine angle tumour).

FACIAL NERVE (VII)

AETIOLOGY

- **Idiopathic**: Bell's palsy.

> ## MICRO-facts
>
> ### Bell's palsy
>
> - The most common cause of a lower motor neuron pattern of facial nerve weakness.
>   - Rapid onset of weakness, peaking at 1–2 days. May be complete paralysis.
>   - Onset may be preceded by aching around ear/mastoid.
> - Thought to be a post-viral phenomenon.
> - Bell's palsy is a diagnosis of exclusion.
> - Management:
>   - A short course of oral **steroids** has been shown to improve the prognosis for recovery.
>   - The use of **acyclovir** is controversial but may be beneficial early in the disease course.
>   - Eye care is important to prevent eye damage as the cornea will be exposed.
> - Most patients make a full recovery, but some individuals will have residual facial weakness.

- **Neoplastic**:
  - parotid gland tumour;
  - cerebellopontine angle tumours.
- **Vascular**
- **Inflammatory/infective**:
  - sarcoidosis;
  - Ramsay Hunt syndrome (herpes zoster affecting the geniculate ganglion; characteristic sign is vesicles around external auditory meatus);
  - basal meningitis;
  - Lyme disease.
- **Trauma**: fracture of the base of the skull.

CLINICAL FEATURES

- Weakness of the intrinsic muscles of the face on the side of the affected nerve.
  - **Upper motor neuron lesion**: sparing of forehead muscles due to bilateral upper motor neuron innervation.
  - **Lower motor neuron lesion**: complete facial weakness, **including** forehead.
- Disruption to taste sensation in the anterior two-thirds of the tongue on the affected side.
- **Hyperacusis**: The VII nerve also supplies stapedius in the middle ear, which acts to dampen noise.
- Pain behind the ear: The VII nerve supplies a small patch of sensation over the pinna of the ear.

VESTIBULOCOCHLEAR NERVE (VIII)

- See Section 7.4.

LOWER CRANIAL NERVES

- The lower cranial nerves (e.g. the glossopharyngeal [IX], vagus [X], spinal accessory [XI] and hypoglossal [XII] nerves) are often affected together due to their close anatomical relation (see **Table 6.1**).
- May be affected in bulbar or pseudobulbar palsy, which is a feature of numerous conditions (see **Table 6.2**).

Table 6.2 **Bulbar and pseudobulbar palsy**

PSEUDOBULBAR PALSY	BULBAR PALSY
Disturbance of the corticobulbar pathways to cranial nerves V, VII, X, XI and XII	Bilateral disturbance of the IX, X and XII cranial nerves
Emotional lability	No emotional lability
Spastic tongue	Tongue wasting and fasiculations
Brisk gag reflex and jaw jerk	Normal/diminished reflexes
Nasal speech	Slow and 'thick' speech
Causes: Vascular: bilateral infarctions Inflammatory Malignancy: high brainstem tumours, may have bilateral symptoms Degeneration: motor neuron disease, PSP, MSA	**Causes:** Motor neuron disease Syringobulbia Inflammatory: Guillan–Barré and acute intermittent porphyria Infective: poliomyelitis and Lyme disease Myasthenia gravis

MSA, multiple system atrophy; PSP, progressive supranuclear palsy.

Neurological zones

AETIOLOGY

- Bulbar or pseudobulbar palsy.
- Isolated or ipsilateral nerve palsies:
  - **vascular**;
  - **inflammatory/infective**;
  - **malignancy**: tumour affecting the jugular foramen (e.g. glomus jugulare tumour);
  - **trauma**: base-of-skull fracture.

CLINICAL FEATURES

- **Glossopharyngeal nerve palsy**:
  - dysphagia: affecting solids and liquids equally;
  - dysarthria;
  - gag reflex: may be diminished or normal;
  - loss of taste sensation on the posterior third of the tongue.
- **Vagus nerve palsy**:
  - dysphagia: affecting solids and liquids equally;
  - dysarthria;
  - unilateral X nerve palsy;
  - asymmetry of the soft palate;
  - uvula deviation away from the side of the lesion;
  - failure of elevation of the soft palate;
  - autonomic symptoms: due to loss of parasympathetic tone.
- **Spinal accessory nerve palsy**:
  - weakness of the trapezius muscle: inability to raise the ipsilateral shoulder;
  - weakness of the sternocleidomastoid muscle: weakness of head turning towards the opposite side.
- **Hypoglossal nerve palsy**:
  - dysarthria;
  - tongue wasting and fasciculations;
  - unilateral lesion: tongue deviates towards the side of lesion.

6.3 BRAINSTEM INFARCTION

- The brainstem is affected in stroke due to posterior circulation dysfunction. Several distinct syndromes exist (see Section 3.7 MICRO-print).

6.4 BRAINSTEM DEATH

- Damage to the cardiac and respiratory centres of the medulla rendering the patient irreversibly unconscious. Respiration and circulation may be artificially maintained, but the patient is pronounced dead when four certain criteria are met:

1. A known pathology causing significant and irreversible brain damage.
2. Any reversible causes of reduced consciousness are corrected (including metabolic, endocrine and circulatory disturbances; the effects of drugs and core temperature).
3. The patient must have ceased spontaneous breathing and require mechanical ventilation (in the absence of anaesthetic agents).
4. The effects of any neuromuscular drugs should have worn off.

- Once these preconditions are fulfilled, the brainstem reflexes should be examined. These tests should be carried out by two experienced doctors, at least one of whom must be a consultant, and should be performed on two separate occasions.
  - Fixed pupils (unresponsive to light).
  - Absent corneal reflex.
  - Vestibular-ocular reflex absent: Absence of eye movements after slow injection of more than 50 ml ice-cold water into each ear.
  - No motor response.
  - No gag reflex.
  - No cough reflex: in response to bronchial stimulation by a suction catheter being passed down an endotracheal tube.
  - No respiratory effort in response to a pCO_2 of 6.5 kPa.

MICRO-case

Bell's palsy

A 43-year-old female hairdresser visits the emergency department. She noticed the left side of her face was droopy. When she took a drink, the water trickled out of the left side of her mouth. She is concerned that she may have had a stroke.

She complains of earache and reports her regular Chinese take-away tasted different from normal. She has had no recent fevers that she can remember and does not complain of any limb weakness, headaches or visual disturbance.

On examination, there is a left-sided facial droop, and she is unable to smile, blow out her cheeks effectively, close her eye completely or wrinkle her forehead on the left side. Her facial sensation is normal. There are no other neurological abnormalities. On further examination you notice a painful vesicular rash in the auditory canal.

Ramsay Hunt syndrome is diagnosed. The patient is given a reducing dose of prednisolone and a course of aciclovir for 1 week. She is also instructed to tape her eye closed overnight and is prescribed some artificial tears to prevent corneal abrasion.

continued...

Neurological zones

continued...

You ask her to see her general practitioner in 2 weeks for a review and advise her that most patients with Bell's palsy make a good recovery, but it often takes time.

Summary points

- Many patients with a facial nerve palsy are brought to the emergency department (ED) with a suspected stroke.
- It is vital to give eye care advice to patients with Bell's palsy as corneal abrasion can occur, which could compromise vision.
- Steroids are used in Bell's palsy as they are thought to hasten recovery. Patients should be started on a high dose for 5 days.
- Recovery from Bell's palsy can often take a long time, and it may not be complete.

6.5 CEREBELLAR DISEASE

Clinical features

- Symptoms of cerebellar disease are common to all cerebellar disorders.
- In general, cerebellar disease produces ipsilateral symptoms.
- **Ataxia**:
  - Impairment of the coordination of movement:
    - unilateral cerebellar disease: patients veer towards the side of the lesion;
    - bilateral cerebellar disease: broad-based unsteady gait.
  - Romberg's test is normal (no evidence of **sensory** ataxia).
- **Intention tremor**:
  - Manifestation of ataxia affecting the limbs – tremor worsens on purposeful movement due to impaired coordination of movement.
  - The patient may display past pointing with overshooting of the target.
- **Dysdiadochokinesis**:
  - Lack of coordination in performing a rapidly alternating repetitive task – due to difficulty in coordinating antagonistic muscle groups.
- **Nystagmus**:
  - Inability to coordinate eye movements.
  - Classical nystagmus of cerebellar disease is a horizontal jerk nystagmus:
    - worse on looking towards the side of the lesion;
    - fast phase directed towards the side of the lesion.
- **Dysarthria**:
  - usually slurred (as if drunk);
  - may be described as 'scanning' with explosive variations in intensity.
- **Hypotonia**

MICRO-print

Ataxia-telangiectasia

- Autosomal recessive inherited ataxic disorder due to mutations in the *ATM* gene. Normally, the protein product of this gene is involved in DNA repair.
- Presents with cerebellar dysfunction in infancy in combination with immunodeficiency and telangiectasia over the eyes and skin in sun-exposed areas.
- Magnetic resonance imaging (MRI) of the brain will show cerebellar atrophy. Alpha-fetoprotein is elevated, and immunoglobulin (Ig) electrophoresis will reveal low serum IgA and IgE. Genetic testing is diagnostic.
- There is no disease-modifying therapy; antibiotics should be used to treat infections, but death usually occurs in adolescence. Genetic counselling should be offered to family members.
- Prognosis is poor; affected individuals become immobile within 5 years of onset.

MICRO-facts

Symptoms of cerebellar disease

Can easily be remembered by the mnemonic DANISH:

D → Dysdiadochokinesis
A → Ataxia
N → Nystagmus
I → Intention tremor
S → Scanning speech
H → Hypotonia

AETIOLOGY

- **Vascular**: infarction and haemorrhage.
- **Space-occupying lesions**:
  - metastases or primary neoplasms;
  - hydrocephalus.
- **Drugs**: especially alcohol; medications such as anticonvulsants (especially phenytoin) and benzodiazepines.
- **Infections**:
  - bacterial meningitis, especially *Hemophilus influenzae* infection in children;
  - viral meningoencephalitis;
  - brain abscess (the cerebellum is the site to 10–20% of brain abscesses).

Neurological zones

- **Inflammatory**:
  - multiple sclerosis;
  - paraneoplastic antibodies, particularly in ovarian and breast cancer (see Section 20.2).
- **Wernicke's encephalopathy**: (see Section 20.5).
- **Inherited disorders**:
  - ataxia telangectasia;
  - inherited spinocerebellar ataxias (SCAs) (e.g. Friedrich's ataxia).
- Multisystem atrophy, cerebellar type.
- Structural abnormalities (e.g. syringobulbia, Arnold–Chiari malformation).
- Vitamin E deficiency.
- Hyper- or hypothyroidism.

MICRO-print

Friedriech's ataxia

- Inherited ataxic disorder with neurological and cardiac features. Most common spinocerebellar ataxia.
- Autosomal dominant defect in the gene that encodes a protein called frataxin, which is involved in iron metabolism.
- The spinocerebellar tracts, dorsal columns and corticospinal tracts within the spinal cord are all affected. In addition, there is degeneration of myelinated peripheral nerves.
- Average age of clinical features is 11 years, with:
  - cerebellar dysfunction and pyramidal tract dysfunction: impairment of touch and proprioception and a peripheral neuropathy;
  - pes cavus;
  - upgoing plantars in the presence of absent ankle reflexes;
  - 75% of patients with hypertrophic cardiomyopathy and musculoskeletal deformity.
- Genetic testing is diagnostic. Additional investigations may include MRI brain/spinal cord and nerve conduction studies, as well as cardiac investigations.
  - Vitamin E deficiency should be excluded, as the presentation can be very similar.
- Management is primarily supportive:
  - Antioxidant drugs such as idebenone can produce some benefit.
  - Cardiomyopathy should be managed in the normal way.
  - Genetic counselling should be offered to the patient and family members.

MICRO-print

Arnold–Chiari malformation

- A developmental abnormality in which the cerebellar tonsils herniate through the foramen magnum into the cervical spinal canal:
  - Compression of the brainstem and cerebellum can affect cranial nerves, the cerebellum and ascending/descending tracts.
  - In addition, blockage of the flow of CSF can produce a non-communicating hydrocephalus, and chronically it will lead to swelling of the central canal with the development of syringobulbia.
- Patients present with symptoms of raised ICP or neurological deficit, including cerebellar dysfunction.
- MRI brain is diagnostic.
- Surgical intervention, including high-cervical laminectomy or suboccipital craniectomy or shunt insertion.

INVESTIGATIONS

- **MRI brain**: to identify a vascular or structural lesion in the posterior fossa or features of demyelination.
- **Blood investigations**:
  - autoimmune screen;
  - paraneoplastic antibodies.
- Lumbar puncture for CSF examination.

MICRO-case

Cerebellar infarction

A 57-year-old man presents to the emergency department with a 4-hour history of severe dizziness, accompanied by nausea and vomiting and difficulty walking. His wife also reports that she has noticed that his speech has become difficult to understand, and that he is falling to the left side when trying to walk. He denies headache or visual disturbance and does not have any sensory changes or pain. His hearing is normal. He has never had any previous similar episodes, but had an episode of transient right-sided visual loss 2 years ago. He has a past medical history of hypertension and hypercholesterolaemia, for which he is on medication. He is also a smoker.

On examination, he is alert with a Glasgow Coma Scale (GCS) score of 15/15. His heart rhythm is noted to be irregularly irregular.

continued...

continued...

There is marked nystagmus, with the fast phase towards the left, but the pupillary reflexes are normal. Speech is jerky. A coarse intention tremor is present on the left side, which is revealed by finger-nose and heel-shin testing. Neurological examination is normal on the right side. There is no limb weakness, and the reflexes are normal. Sensation appears to be intact throughout. On standing, examination reveals a wide-based gait, with stumbling to the left. Romberg's test is negative.

Blood investigations are normal, but MRI scanning reveals a small area of low attenuation in the left cerebellar hemisphere, and the diagnosis of cerebellar infarction is made. An electrocardiogram (ECG) reveals that the patient is in atrial fibrillation.

The patient is unsuitable for thrombolytic therapy and is started on secondary prevention. Over the next few weeks, his ataxia and dizziness improve. Following extensive physiotherapy input, he is eventually discharged with minimal residual features. He is started on oral anticoagulation to reduce the risk of further ischaemic events.

Summary points

- The distribution of ataxia and characteristics of nystagmus allow localisation of a cerebellar lesion.
- Patents who have a cerebellar lesion may demonstrate normal limb power but have lost function due to ataxia.
- An MRI brain scan is preferable to computed tomography (CT) for imaging of the posterior fossa.

7 Vestibular system

7.1 OVERVIEW

- Orientation of the body requires input from three sensory systems: vision, proprioception and the **vestibular** system.
- The vestibular system has two main components:
  - **Semicircular canals**: three endolymph-containing structures that detect rotational movement;
  - **Otoliths**: two structures (utricle and saccule) that detect acceleration; contain otoconia (small particles that stimulate hair cells due to inertial movement).
- Damage to the vestibular apparatus or the vestibular nerve leads to a mismatch between vestibular input and that from other sensory systems; this leads to an inappropriate sensation of movement, called **vertigo**.
  - Compensation for this mismatch occurs over weeks and symptoms disappear.
  - If the vestibular system is damaged, loss of input from an intact sensory system (e.g. closing eyes) will increase the sensation of vertigo.
- **Nystagmus** (see Section 1.5) is a common feature of vestibular disease. Uncontrolled eye movements occur due to a false sensation of head movement.
- Vestibular disorders are commonly due to vestibulocochlear (VIII) nerve damage; they may involve only the vestibular branch or may also affect the cochlear nerve, producing **hearing loss** or **tinnitus**.
- Damage to the central connections of the vestibular system in the brainstem may also occur; this causes **central vestibular dysfunction**.

7.2 BENIGN PAROXYSMAL POSITIONAL VERTIGO

DEFINITION

- Benign paroxysmal positional vertigo (BPPV) is vertigo caused by abnormal particulate matter in the semicircular canals.

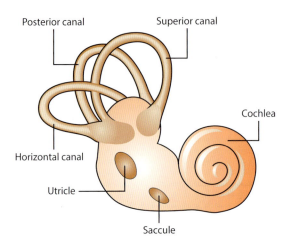

Fig. 7.1 Diagram of the semicircular canals and cochlea.

PATHOPHYSIOLOGY

- Normally, the semicircular canals detect motion of the head via displacement of the cupula due to movement of the endolymph within the central canal.
- The presence of particulate matter within the canal interferes with this process and produces abnormal sensations of movement:
  - Particulate matter commonly consists of otoconia displaced from the utricle. See **Fig. 7.1**.

EPIDEMIOLOGY

- **Age**: rare in patients under 35 years, unless precipitated by head trauma.
- Other risk factors include viral labyrinthitis, inner ear surgery and Ménière's disease.

CLINICAL FEATURES

- Vertigo triggered by head movement.
  - May be associated with nausea and loss of balance.
  - Symptoms may resolve after a period of time or occur in an episodic fashion.
- Nystagmus (see the following MICRO-print).

MICRO-print

Nystagmus in BPPV

- Positional.
- There is 5- to 10-second delay prior to onset after head movement; lasts for 5–30 seconds.

continued...

---

continued...

- Visual fixation does not suppress nystagmus.
- If only the posterior canal is involved, the nystagmus will be purely rotational. If only the horizontal canal is involved, the nystagmus will be purely horizontal.
- Repeated Dix–Hallpike manoeuvres cause the nystagmus to fatigue or disappear temporarily.

INVESTIGATIONS

- **Dix–Hallpike** (also referred to as the Nylen–Barany) manoeuvre (see **Fig. 7.2**). A positive test occurs when vertigo and nystagmus are induced.
- **Audiogram**: to exclude vestibulocochlear nerve pathology.
- **Magnetic resonance imaging (MRI) of the brain**: to detect structural lesions of the vestibulocochlear nerve.

MANAGEMENT

- **Canalith repositioning manoeuvres**: specific movements of the patient's head results in repositioning of debris from the semicircular canal to the utricle where it can be reabsorbed (e.g. Epley manoeuver, Sermont liberatory manoeuvre).
  - The Dix–Hallpike manoeuvre should be performed afterwards to check whether the treatment has been effective.
- **Surgery**: may be required in patients with symptoms that have not resolved spontaneously and where canalith repositioning manoeuvres have been ineffective.
- No evidence to support use of vestibulosuppressants.

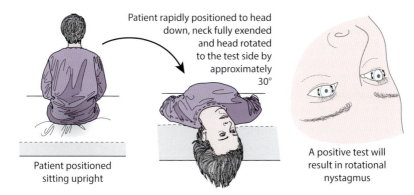

Patient rapidly positioned to head down, neck fully exended and head rotated to the test side by approximately 30°

Patient positioned sitting upright

A positive test will result in rotational nystagmus

Fig. 7.2 Dix–Hallpike manoeuvre.

Neurological zones

7.3 MÉNIÈRE'S DISEASE (IDIOPATHIC ENDOLYMPHATIC HYDROPS)

DEFINITION

- Inner ear disorder resulting in a triad of vertigo, hearing loss and tinnitus.

AETIOLOGY

- Usually idiopathic.
- May occur secondary to increased production or reduced reabsorption of endolymph: trauma, electrolyte imbalance or infection.
- Rarely may be familial, related to mutations in the cochlin gene.

PATHOPHYSIOLOGY

- Endolymph is a potassium-rich solution; perilymph is potassium depleted. Normally, vestibular nerve receptors are bathed in endolymph, but mixing with perilymph will reduce the local potassium concentration and disrupt vestibular function.
- Increased pressure within the endolymph may cause an acute rupture in the separation between the endolymph and perilymph.

EPIDEMIOLOGY

- Peak incidence is in individuals aged 20–50 years.

CLINICAL FEATURES

- Characterised by episodic symptoms occurring at intervals of weeks to years.
- Sensorineural hearing loss, vertigo, tinnitus and a feeling of aural fullness; vertigo associated with nystagmus and nausea.
  - Recovery usually occurs after minutes to days.
  - Many patients make a full recovery between attacks; others note a progressive deterioration in hearing and vestibular function.

INVESTIGATIONS

- Diagnosis is usually clinical, but if there is diagnostic doubt, further investigation may be useful:
  - **Audiometry**: demonstrates a characteristic pattern of sensorineural hearing loss mainly affecting low frequencies.
  - **Brain imaging**: MRI brain scan may be useful to exclude a cerebellopontine angle tumour, particularly if symptoms are unilateral.

MANAGEMENT

- Treat any underlying cause.
- Symptomatic treatment:
  - Vestibulosuppressants (e.g. prochlorperazine for symptomatic relief of vertigo);
  - Steroids to suppress inflammation associated with attacks;
  - Betahistine (histamine agonist).
- Reduce the frequency of attacks:
  - Avoid any notable triggers. This often includes one or more dietary components.
  - Diuretics (e.g. hydrochlorthiazide, acetazolamide) appear to reduce the pressure of the endolymph and reduce the frequency of attacks.
  - Steroids and betahistine are partially effective as prophylaxis.
- Selective chemical labyrinthectomy: used in severe cases. Gentamicin is infused into inner ear resulting in vestibular damage (hearing is usually retained).
- **Surgery** may be attempted in severe, medically intractable disease – endolymphatic sac decompression, division of vestibular nerve or total labyrinthectomy.

PROGNOSIS

- Of Ménière's sufferers, 60–80% do not ever develop permanent disability; a minority will develop permanent sensorineural hearing loss or vestibular dysfunction.

7.4 VESTIBULAR NEURONITIS AND LABYRINTHITIS

DEFINITION

- **Vestibular neuronitis**: acute deficit of the peripheral vestibular system resulting in vertigo, nystagmus, nausea and vomiting.
- **Labyrinthitis**: acute inflammation of the inner ear resulting in hearing loss and tinnitus in addition to vestibular dysfunction.

PATHOPHYSIOLOGY

- **Vestibular neuronitis**: appears to involve disruption of the neural connection between the vestibular organ and the central nervous system (CNS). In some cases, a reactivation of latent herpes simplex virus type 1 is implicated.
- **Labyrinthitis**: may be caused by either viral (including rarely the Ramsay Hunt syndrome) or bacterial infection or an autoimmune process.

CLINICAL FEATURES

- Acute vestibular dysfunction.
- Labyrinthitis also involves cochlear dysfunction, leading to hearing loss and tinnitus.

MICRO-print

Clinical differentiation of central and peripheral causes of vestibular dysfunction

- It is important to differentiate isolated vestibular failure in vestibular neuronitis from central causes of vestibular dysfunction, which may present similarly but have different management.
- Central vestibular dysfunction is most often caused by brainstem infarction or multiple sclerosis.
- Nystagmus: skew deviation (i.e. upward movement of both eyes in different directions) is specific for **central dysfunction**.
- Head thrust test (passive movement of the head and neck to the left or right while asking a subject to focus his or her gaze on a distant object): Failure to maintain fixation and the observation of correctionary saccadic eye movements suggests **peripheral vestibular dysfunction**.

INVESTIGATIONS

- **Brain imaging**: MRI head with or without diffusion-weighted imaging will exclude a central cause of vestibular dysfunction.
- Further investigations may be needed to determine the cause of labyrinthitis:
  - Most cases are viral.
  - Further investigations (including cerebrospinal fluid [CSF] analysis) may be necessary to exclude bacterial infection.
  - Autoimmune labyrinthitis is defined by a response to a trial of steroid therapy.

MANAGEMENT

- Primarily supportive with rehydration, anti-emetics and vestibulosuppressants.
- Bacterial or autoimmune labyrinthitis will require antibiotics or steroids, respectively.

PROGNOSIS

- Spontaneous recovery almost always occurs within 6 weeks.

MICRO-case

Benign paroxysmal positional vertigo

A 49-year-old civil servant presents to her general practitioner (GP) with 'dizziness'. The symptoms have been present for the past week, and they are not improving. The bouts of vertigo are intermittent, lasting up to 1 minute each time, and come on when moving her head. They are not present when she keeps her head still. She has had some associated nausea and has vomited once. She also complains of being slightly unsteady on her feet during the attacks of vertigo. There are no symptoms of tinnitus or hearing loss.

On examination, she has rotary nystagmus, and the Dix–Hallpike manoeuvre is positive. She has no other focal neurological signs.

The diagnosis of BPPV is made.

Epley's manoeuvre is performed, and the patient makes a good recovery.

Summary points

- BPPV is common.
- Diagnosis and treatment are mainly clinical; further invasive treatments are seldom needed.
- Patients are likely to have recurrent episodes of BPPV.

8 Visual tracts

8.1 ANATOMY AND PHYSIOLOGY

- Nerve impulses generated by the action of light on the photoreceptors of the retina are carried to the primary visual cortex (see Section 3.5) by the optic (II) nerve.
- The optic chiasm allows the right and left visual fields to be separated. The signal carried by the optic nerve anterior to the chiasm is monocular; the signal carried by the optic tract posterior to the chiasm is binocular but represents only one side of visual space.
- Outflow from V1 takes place in two parallel streams with different specialization:
    - The **ventral** stream is concerned with detail, colour and object recognition.
    - The **dorsal** stream is concerned with movement and contrast.
- Visual loss or disturbance may occur due to pathology at any point in the visual tracts; the pattern of visual loss suggests the location of the lesion.
- See **Fig. 8.1**.

8.2 PATTERNS OF VISUAL LOSS

MONOCULAR VISUAL LOSS

AETIOLOGY

- Occurs if a lesion affects the eye itself or the optic nerve anterior to the optic chiasm.
- **Vascular** pathology affecting the eye/optic nerve:
    - amaurosis fugax (see Section 12.2 – MICRO-facts: Features of TIA);
    - anterior ischaemic optic neuritis (see Section 21.1);
    - retinal vein thrombosis;
    - retinal arterial thrombosis.
- **Optic neuropathy (ON)**, which can be:
    - structural (e.g. tumour);
    - inflammatory (e.g. multiple sclerosis).

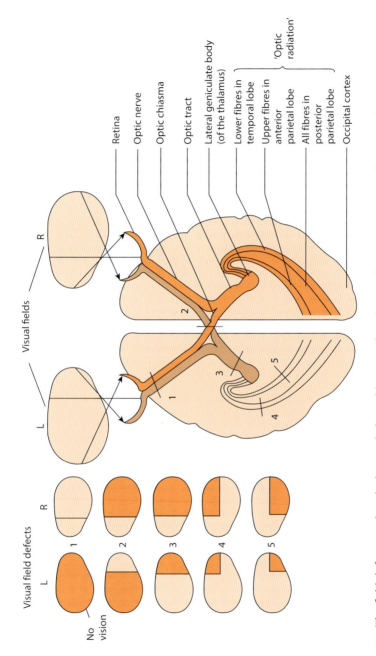

Fig. 8.1 The field defects produced when pathological lesions effect the visual tract. Note that information from the right side of each retina passes to the right side of the brain and vice versa.

- **Inflammatory disorders**: scleritis/episcleritis, uveitis.
- **Ocular disorders**: cataracts, glaucoma, retinal detachment, trauma, macular degeneration.

INVESTIGATIONS

- Ophthalmoscopy and slit-lamp examination. In typical ON, retinal examination is normal because the inflammation lies behind the optic nerve head (see Section 8.3).
- Magnetic resonance imaging (MRI) of the orbit may identify structural disease. MRI brain may reveal evidence of central nervous system (CNS) demyelination, which offers useful prognostic information; ON plus demyelination on MRI means subsequent risk of multiple sclerosis is approximately 70%.
- Visual evoked potentials may be used to identify a lesion of the optic nerve.

MANAGEMENT

- Dependent on cause.

BINOCULAR VISUAL LOSS

DEFINITIONS

- See **Fig. 8.1**;
- Hemianopia: half of the visual field affected;
- Quadrantanopia: quadrant/quarter of the visual field affected;
- Bitemporal hemianopia: both temporal fields affected;
- Homonymous hemianopia: one side of the visual field affected (e.g. left temporal field and right nasal field). Result of lesions posterior to the optic chiasm.

AETIOLOGY

- Occurs with damage to the visual tracts at or after the optic chiasm.
- **Structural lesions** (e.g. tumour, abscess, aneurysm):
  - Pituitary tumours and craniopharyngiomas classically cause compression of the optic chiasm, resulting in bitemporal hemianopia (see **Fig. 8.1** and Section 13.5).
    - The nerve fibres representing the temporal visual fields decussate at the chiasm and lie medially; compression from a tumour affects these fibres first.
- **Vascular lesions**:
  - A posterior circulation ischaemic stroke will cause a homonymous hemianopia.
  - Infarction of the lateral geniculate nucleus will produce a homonymous hemianopia, but compared to a cortical stroke, it will be markedly different in each eye (incongruent).

Neurological zones

- Infarction of the optic radiation can produce a homonymous quadrantanopia; fibres in the parietal lobe carry information from the inferior visual field, and fibres in the temporal lobe (Meyer's loop) carry information from the superior visual field.

8.3 OPTIC NERVE DISORDERS

PAPILLOEDEMA

DEFINITION

- Swelling of the optic disc due to raised intracranial pressure (ICP).

AETIOLOGY

- Raised ICP due to:
  - mass lesions such as tumours;
  - intracranial haemorrhage;
  - infection, including meningitis and encephalitis;
  - venous sinus thrombosis;
  - idiopathic intracranial hypertension.

CLINICAL FEATURES

- Vision is often unaffected by papilloedema, but enlargement of the blind spot may occur.
- Papilloedema is typically binocular. If present in one eye, it is more likely to be papillitis (see the following section on optic neuritis) or drusen (retinal deposits).
- Other symptoms related to the underlying cause.

MANAGEMENT

- Treat the underlying cause.
- Surgical decompression of the optic nerve sheath may be appropriate if the ICP cannot be reduced.

OPTIC NEURITIS

DEFINITION

- Inflammation of the optic nerve.

AETIOLOGY

- **Demyelination**, associated with multiple sclerosis, is the most common cause. Also occurs in neuromyelitis optica.
- **Infection**, including viral encephalitis, infectious mononucleosis and herpes zoster
- **Inflammation**: granulomatous (tuberculosis, sarcoidosis) or local (sinusitis).

- Idiopathic.
- Nutritional deficiency/toxins (e.g. B$_{12}$ or alcohol).
- Leber's hereditary ON (see MICRO-print, Leber's optic neuropathy)

MICRO-print

Nutritional deficiency/toxic optic neuropathy

- Certain toxins or nutritional deficiencies can cause optic neuropathy.
- Patients usually present with a slow onset of loss of their central visual field in the context of malnutrition and chronic alcohol excess.
- Papilloedema may be apparent in the acute phase; later, optic atrophy develops.
- Treatment is with cessation of alcohol consumption and replacement of vitamins, particularly vitamin B$_{12}$.
- Other causes include lead and the anti-tuberculous medications ethambutol and isoniazid.

MICRO-print

Leber's optic neuropathy

- Caused by a mutation of mitochondrial DNA.
- Mainly affects men, but the gene is passed to all offspring of a female carrier.
- Presents with painless loss of the central visual field in early adulthood.
- Initially monocular, but the other eye is involved later.
- In the acute phase, affected eyes will display an appearance similar to papilloedema but without true optic disc oedema (the two can be distinguished by fluoroscein angiography).
- Optic atrophy develops later.
- Currently, no disease-modifying treatment is available. Genetic counselling should be offered to family members.

CLINICAL FEATURES

- Monocular visual loss that progresses over hours to days; severity of visual loss is highly variable.
- Eye pain is common and occurs mainly on eye movement.
- Relative afferent papillary defect (RAPD) on the affected side (see Section 2.2, Optic Nerve).
- Ophthalmoscopy:
    - May show **papillitis** (optic disc swelling due to inflammation of the optic nerve head).

- May be normal if the inflammation is behind the optic nerve head (**retrobulbar neuritis**).
- Optic neuritis can cause optic atrophy, which manifests as a pale optic disc.

INVESTIGATIONS

- Diagnosis of optic neuritis is usually clinical.
- A patient presenting with optic neuritis must be investigated for CNS demyelination and subsequent risk for multiple sclerosis.

MICRO-case

Pituitary adenoma

A 40-year-old woman presents to her general practitioner (GP) after noticing that she finds it increasingly difficult to see other cars at crossroads when she is driving. She also reports intermittent headaches over the past 4 weeks, for which she has been taking paracetamol. She denies any double vision or pain on eye movements and is otherwise entirely well. She has no history of cerebrovascular disease or hypertension and is a lifelong non-smoker.

On examination, she has marked bitemporal hemianopia. Examination of the rest of her cranial nerves and peripheral nervous system does not reveal any abnormality, and fundoscopy is normal.

She is seen at the neurology clinic. Blood investigations are normal, but an MRI scan of the brain reveals a pituitary tumour confined to the sella turcica. After review by the neurosurgical team, she is booked for trans-sphenoidal resection of the adenoma, which is performed without complication. Histology confirms the mass to be a pituitary macroadenoma.

She makes a good recovery, and at review 6 weeks later, her bitemporal hemianopia has improved.

Summary points

- The type of visual field defect allows one to identify the likely site of the causative lesion.
- As with other neurological deficits, the speed of onset of visual field symptoms suggests the type of visual tract lesion. Vascular lesions produce rapid deficit, whereas space-occupying lesions tend to be more insidious.

MANAGEMENT

- Intravenous steroids speed recovery but have no effect on disease progression. If visual acuity does not improve, it is important to exclude a structural cause, and plasma exchange can be attempted.

9 Spinal cord

9.1 SPINAL CORD ANATOMY

- The spinal cord extends from the foramen magnum to the conus medullaris at the level of the L2 vertebrae.
- It is composed of numerous white matter tracts (containing nerve axons) surrounding a core of grey matter (containing cell bodies).
- The spinal canal contains cerebrospinal fluid (CSF) and runs down the centre of the cord; it is an extension of the ventricular system within the brain.
- The cord is composed of 31 **spinal segments**; each gives rise to a dorsal (sensory) and ventral (motor) nerve root that combine to form a pair of **spinal nerves**.
    - The segments are named for the vertebrae between which their respective spinal nerves exit the vertebral canal.
- The spinal nerves exit the vertebral canal progressively lower than the spinal segments from which they originate.
    - In the upper cord, spinal nerves exit directly at the level at which they are formed.
    - Further down the cord, the spinal nerves travel down to exit at a lower level (e.g. the spinal nerve exiting between the L2 and L3 vertebrae originates from a spinal segment that actually lies in the thoracic region).
- As the spinal cord finishes at the L2 vertebral level, the spinal nerves of the lower spinal segments form a collection of nerves called the cauda equina.

SENSORY PATHWAYS

- The spinal cord conveys sensory information from the body to the brain via several white matter tracts (see **Figs. 9.1** and **9.2** and **Table 9.1**).
- The area of skin that receives a sensory supply from a single nerve root is called a **dermatome** (see **Fig. 9.3**).

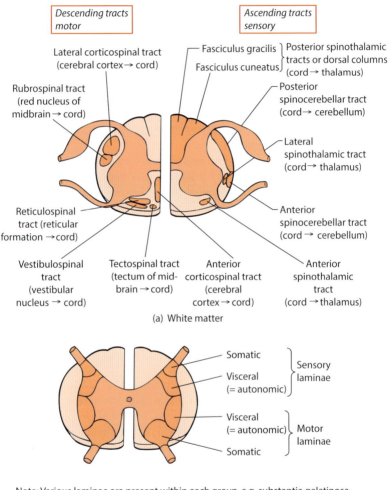

Descending tracts
motor

Ascending tracts
sensory

Lateral corticospinal tract
(cerebral cortex → cord)

Fasciculus gracilis ⎫ Posterior spinothalamic
⎬ tracts or dorsal columns
Fasciculus cuneatus ⎭ (cord → thalamus)

Rubrospinal tract
(red nucleus of
midbrain → cord)

Posterior
spinocerebellar tract
(cord → cerebellum)

Lateral
spinothalamic tract
(cord → thalamus)

Reticulospinal
tract (reticular
formation → cord)

Anterior
spinocerebellar tract
(cord → cerebellum)

Vestibulospinal
tract
(vestibular
nucleus → cord)

Tectospinal tract
(tectum of mid-
brain → cord)

Anterior
corticospinal tract
(cerebral
cortex → cord)

Anterior
spinothalamic
tract
(cord → thalamus)

(a) White matter

Somatic

Visceral
(= autonomic)

⎫
⎬ Sensory
⎭ laminae

Visceral
(= autonomic)

Somatic

⎫
⎬ Motor
⎭ laminae

Note: Various laminae are present within each group, e.g. substantia gelatinosa
within sensory groups

(b) Grey matter

Fig. 9.1 Diagram of the spinal cord in cross section with dorsal columns,
spinothalamic tracts, central canal and anterior white commissure.

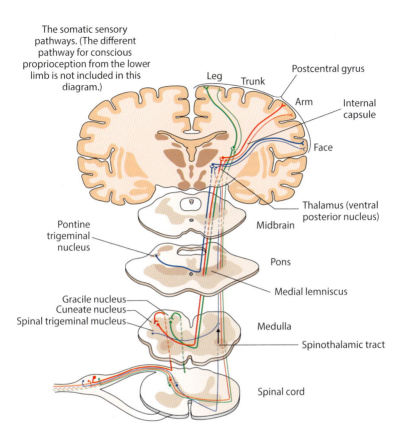

The somatic sensory pathways. (The different pathway for conscious proprioception from the lower limb is not included in this diagram.)

Leg Trunk

Postcentral gyrus

Arm

Internal capsule

Face

Thalamus (ventral posterior nucleus)

Midbrain

Pontine trigeminal nucleus

Pons

Medial lemniscus

Gracile nucleus
Cuneate nucleus
Spinal trigeminal mucleus

Medulla

Spinothalamic tract

Spinal cord

Fig. 9.2 Schematic of the spinothalamic and dorsal column systems showing points of decussation and levels of synapse.

Table 9.1 Ascending spinal tracts

	SPINOTHALAMIC TRACT	DORSAL COLUMNS
Sensory modalities	Pain and temperature	Fine touch, proprioception
Site of decussation	Level of entry to the spinal cord (via the anterior white commissure)	Medulla
Topographic map	Rostral structures (e.g. arms) represented medially; caudal structures (e.g. legs) represented laterally; relatively imprecise topographic map	Caudal structures represented medially; rostral structures represented laterally; precise topographic map maintained

Neurological zones

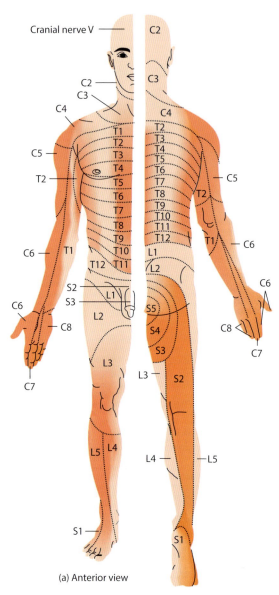

(a) Anterior view

(b) Posterior view

Fig. 9.3 Diagram of dermatomes supplied by each spinal cord root.

MOTOR PATHWAYS

- Motor information from the brain is conveyed to muscles via several tracts, most importantly the **corticospinal tract**, whose fibres decussate at the medullary pyramids in the brainstem (therefore also known as the **pyramidal tracts**), producing crossed motor representation of the body in the motor cortex.
- See **Fig. 9.4**.
- Each spinal nerve root provides a motor supply to a particular muscle group (a **myotome**):
  - **shoulder**: C5, abduction; C7, adduction;
  - **elbow**: C5–C6, flexion; C7–C8, extension; C6, pronation/supination;
  - **wrist**: C6–C7, flexion/extension;
  - **fingers**: C7–C8, flexion/extension; T1, abduction/adduction;

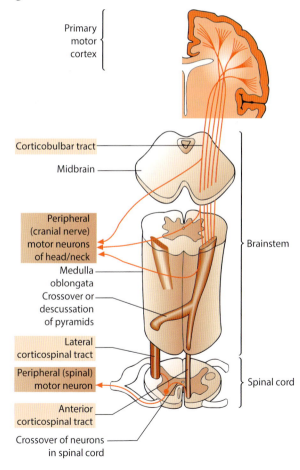

Primary motor cortex

Corticobulbar tract

Midbrain

Peripheral (cranial nerve) motor neurons of head/neck

Medulla oblongata

Crossover or descussation of pyramids

Lateral corticospinal tract

Peripheral (spinal) motor neuron

Anterior corticospinal tract

Crossover of neurons in spinal cord

Brainstem

Spinal cord

Fig. 9.4 Schematic of the pyramidal tract showing points of decussation and synapse.

- **hip**: L2–L3, flexion and adduction; L4–L5, extension and abduction;
- **knee**: L3–L4, extension; L5–S1, flexion;
- **ankle**: L4–L5, dorsiflexion; S1–S2, plantar flexion.
- Each reflex of the upper and lower limbs is associated with particular spinal cord roots:
  - triceps: C7;
  - biceps: C5–C6;
  - brachioradialis: C6;
  - patellar: L4;
  - Achilles: S1–S2.

> ## MICRO-facts
>
> Damage to the **pyramidal tract** at any point produces a particular pattern of weakness with **extensors weaker than flexors** in the upper limbs and **extensors stronger than flexors** in the lower limbs. This is illustrated by the classic resting position of a stroke patient with the arm held in flexion and the leg held in extension.

AUTONOMIC PATHWAYS (SEE FIG. 9.5)

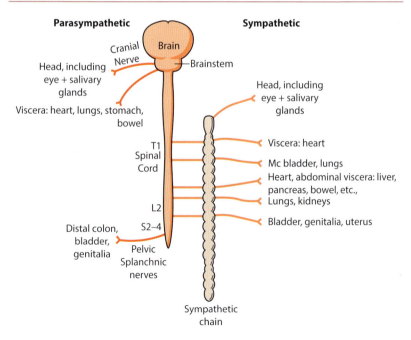

Fig. 9.5 Diagram of the autonomic supply with sympathetic and parasympathetic centres.

- **Sympathetic innervation** arises from the spinal cord between T1 and L2.
- **Parasympathetic innervation**: from cranial nerves and sacral nerve roots:
  - Cranial nerves (especially the vagus [X] nerve) supply all intrathoracic structures and intra-abdominal structures up to two-thirds of the way along the transverse colon.
  - Sacral spinal roots (S2–S3) innervate the remainder of the gastrointestinal tract as well as other pelvic structures.

SPINAL CORD BLOOD SUPPLY (SEE FIG. 9.6)

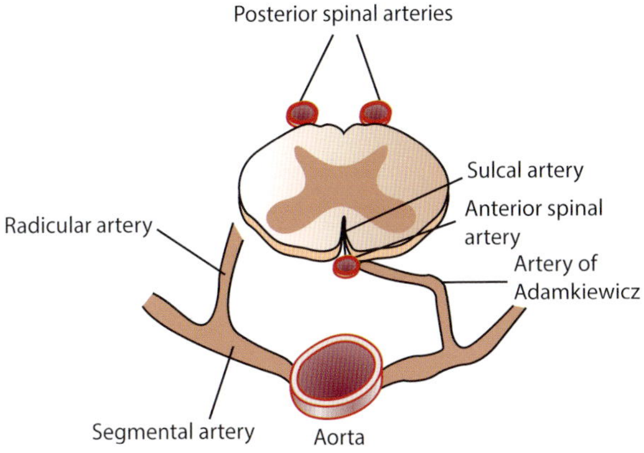

Fig. 9.6 Diagram of spinal cord blood supply, including anterior and posterior spinal arteries.

- The anterior and posterior spinal arteries are branches of the vertebral arteries.
- They are supplemented by collateral supply from the (anterior and posterior) radicular arteries, which are indirect branches of the descending aorta.
- The artery of Adamkiewicz is an enlarged radicular artery in the lumbar region, usually on the left, which anastomoses with the anterior spinal artery. Infarction of this artery can lead to paraplegia.

9.2 ANTERIOR SPINAL ARTERY OCCLUSION

PATHOPHYSIOLOGY

- The cervical cord has poor collateral supply; occlusion of the anterior spinal artery produces ischaemia/infarction of the anterior two-thirds of the cord.
- The **dorsal columns** are relatively spared because they receive blood supply from the posterior spinal artery.

AETIOLOGY

- **Vascular**: The vessel may become occluded by atherosclerosis, vasculitis or embolism.

Neurological zones

- **Trauma**.
- **Iatrogenic**: secondary to aortic surgery.
- **Malignancy**: compression of the artery by a tumour.
- **Infection**: meningitis or neurosyphilis.

Clinical features

- Pyramidal tract signs below the level of the lesion (initially flaccid paralysis developing into spasticity).
- Sudden onset back pain.
- Sensory disturbance below the level of the lesion (due to involvement of the spinothalamic tract).
- Fine touch and proprioception preserved as the dorsal columns spared.

Investigations

- **MRI spine**: even with diffusion-weighted imaging (DWI) may not identify an area of infarction because the spinal cord is so narrow but will exclude any structural or compressive lesion.
- Investigations for underlying cause.

Management

- Dependent on the cause of arterial insufficiency:
  - In atherosclerotic disease, secondary prevention should be initiated as for cerebrovascular stroke as well as modification of risk factors.
  - Treatment of underlying disease in other causes.
- Rehabilitation on a dedicated spinal injuries unit.
- Symptomatic treatment similar to that for cerebrovascular stroke.

Prognosis

- Poor; 1 month mortality is about 20–25%.

MICRO-print

Transverse myelitis

- **Inflammation** of the spinal cord that resembles a cord transection but with subacute onset. All of the spinal cord tract can be affected, with a consequent sensory deficit and pyramidal pattern of weakness below the level of the lesion.
- The most common cause is **multiple sclerosis**; other causes include infection and connective tissue disease.
- Investigations: **brain** and **spinal MRI**, viral serology and an autoimmune screen. The presence of demyelinated plaques elsewhere in the central nervous system (CNS) suggests multiple sclerosis.
- **Management** is dependent on the underlying cause; recovery is usual.

9.3 TRAUMATIC SPINAL CORD TRANSECTION

DEFINITION

- Division of the spinal cord due to trauma. Often occurs via anterior dislocation of one vertebra on another or vertebral fracture.

CLINICAL FEATURES

- **Motor features**:
    - initially spinal shock with flaccid paralysis and areflexia;
    - develops into a classical upper motor neuron pattern of weakness with hypertonia, brisk reflexes and upgoing plantars.
- **Sensory features**: complete loss of all modalities below the level of the lesion.
- **Autonomic features** are dependent on level of injury and vary with time:
    - Spinal cord injury above T6 causes **neurogenic shock** due to loss of sympathetic tone to the heart and vasculature.
    - Excessive sympathetic tone develops subsequently due to lack of higher inhibition (hypertension, tachycardia and urge incontinence).
    - Attempted compensation from higher centres can lead to excessive vasodilation above the level of the injury.
- **Respiratory compromise**: Thoracic cord injury may cause denervation of respiratory muscles; transection of cord above C3 will result in apnoea and death if no ventilatory support is available.
- Severity of spinal cord injury can be determined by evaluation of sacral nerve roots:
    - **complete**: absence of anal muscular tone and sensation;
    - **incomplete**: presence of anal muscular tone and sensation plus preservation of some muscular power/sensation below level of lesion.

INVESTIGATIONS

- **MRI spine** will define spinal cord injury but computed tomography (CT) is better at showing bony injury.

MANAGEMENT

- A specialist trauma team, including orthopaedic surgeons/neurosurgeons, should assess the patient as soon as possible, preferably at point of entry to hospital:
    - Spinal immobilisation is used during assessment for injury and instability.
    - Urgent surgical intervention may prevent progression of injury.

Neurological zones

- High-dose corticosteroid in the acute period is shown to reduce oedema and improve prognosis.
- Chronic management of spinal cord injury is primarily supportive:
  - Drugs to reduce spasticity (e.g. baclofen) may help reduce discomfort and improve function in partial transections.
  - Specialist urological management is necessary for incontinence.
- Management by a multidisciplinary team (MDT), including occupational therapists and physiotherapists, is imperative.

PROGNOSIS

- Complete cord transection has very poor prognosis, with less than 5% recovery of function.
- Incomplete injury has a better outlook; with preserved sensory function, there is approximately a 50% chance of the patient being able to walk again.
- There are reductions in life expectancy due to complications related to immobility (e.g. pneumonia and venous thromboembolism).

MICRO-print

Brown-Séquard syndrome

Clinical syndrome resulting from lesion to one-half of spinal cord. Causes include:

- trauma;
- multiple sclerosis;
- spinal cord tumour;
- infection (e.g. tuberculosis).

The clinical features of Brown-Séquard reflect the anatomy:

- Damage to descending tracts that decussate in the brainstem produces **ipsilateral** neurological deficit below the level of the lesion.
- Damage to the corticospinal tract produces upper motor neuron weakness; dorsal column damage will impair the sense of touch as well as proprioception.
- The ascending spinothalamic tract decussates at the point of entering the cord; therefore, pain and temperature are impaired on the **contralateral** side below the level of the lesion.

Treatment and investigation will vary according to the cause of Brown-Séquard syndrome.

9.4 VERTEBRAL DISC PROLAPSE

DEFINITION

- Degeneration of the vertebral disc leading to prolapse and consequent spinal cord or root compression.

PATHOPHYSIOLOGY

- Herniation of the nucleus pulposus (soft core of intervertebral disc) through the annulus fibrosus (fibrous outer shell) may occur due to repeated minor trauma or progressive 'wear and tear':
  - Posteriolateral herniation causes compression of nerve roots as they pass through the intervertebral foramina.
  - Posterior herniation may compress the spinal cord directly.
- Most common in the lumbar area of the spinal cord (95% occur in L4–L5 or L5–S1).

EPIDEMIOLOGY

- **Gender**: males > females.
- **Age**: most common between the ages of 30 and 50 years.
- More common among individuals who perform a lot of manual work involving bending/lifting.

CLINICAL FEATURES

- **Pain**:
  - Often is significant at the site of the lesion.
  - Nerve root compression may cause radiation of pain to the area supplied by the affected root.
  - Radiation of pain from the lumbar region is known as **sciatica**.
- **Neurological deficit**:
  - Compression of a nerve root will result in lower motor neuron weakness and altered sensation in the affected nerve distribution.
  - A prolapse that affects both the spinal cord (myelopathy) and the associated nerve roots (radiculopathy) will produce features of cord damage below the level of the lesion **plus** lower motor neuron weakness at the level of the lesion due to root involvement; this is known as **radiculomyelopathy**.
  - Features of lumbar disc prolapse are different: Prolapse below the L1/L2 vertebral level compresses spinal cord roots only; a central disc prolapse can cause **cauda equina syndrome**:
    - There is lower back pain with radiation down the legs.
    - Sensory loss corresponding to the dermatomes of the compressed roots exists. It is imperative to examine for sensory loss over the perineum, which corresponds to roots S3/S4.
    - There is a lower motor neuron pattern of weakness in the distribution of the compressed roots.
  - Bladder or bowel incontinence occurs if the sacral parasympathetic outflow is affected.

Neurological zones

INVESTIGATIONS

- **Imaging**: Urgent MRI spine is imperative in suspected disc prolapse with motor deficit or bowel and bladder involvement.
  - If neurological deficit is absent, then MRI should only be performed for pain that persists after 6 weeks of conservative management.

MANAGEMENT

- **Neurological deficit present**: Urgent surgical evaluation is necessary as early surgical decompression may minimise progression of symptoms.
- **Neurological deficit absent**: Management should be conservative with physiotherapy and simple analgesia.

9.5 SYRINGOMYELIA

DEFINITION

- Formation of a fluid-filled cavity within the spinal cord known as a syrinx (usually a dilation of the spinal canal).
- When this process occurs in the brainstem, it is known as syringobulbia.

PATHOPHYSIOLOGY

- Syrinx formation is usually related to blockage of the normal flow of CSF with consequent increase in local CSF pressure and dilation of the spinal canal.
- The most common location for a syrinx is the cervical spinal cord.

EPIDEMIOLOGY

- **Age**: onset usually in early adulthood.
- **Prevalence**: 8 cases per 100,000 population (in United States).

AETIOLOGY

- Acquired causes include:
  - trauma;
  - intramedullary tumours;
  - haemorrhage.
- The most common congenital cause is an Arnold–Chiari malformation.

CLINICAL FEATURES

- Dependent on the site of the syrinx and result from compression of adjacent structures.
- Within the cervical cord, the closest tract to the spinal canal is the anterior white commissure, which carries decussating pain and temperature fibres; compression results in:
  - early loss of pain and temperature sensation in a cape distribution (see **Fig. 9.7**);
  - association with pain over the neck and shoulders;

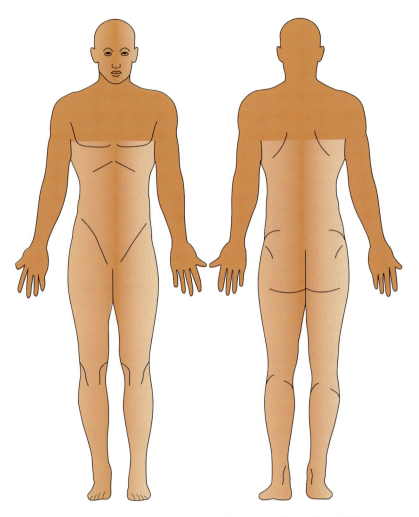

Fig. 9.7 The lesions in this case involves the decussating fibres of the ALS, or spinothalamic tract, for the entire cervical spinal cord. The shaded area shows the cape distribution of sensory loss.

- Further expansion of the syrinx will affect the other spinal cord tracts, producing dorsal column and pyramidal tract deficit below the level of the lesion.
    - This can result in impairing the sense of touch and proprioception at the borders of cape distribution.
- Involvement of nerve roots may produce a lower motor neuron pattern of weakness at the level of the lesion.

INVESTIGATIONS

- **MRI spine** is the investigation of choice to identify a syrinx and any predisposing cause.

MANAGEMENT

- Neurosurgical intervention with decompression or shunt placement may relieve symptoms and prevent progression.
- Any underlying cause of syrinx formation should be resolved if possible to prevent recurrence.

MICRO-print

Spinal cord metastases

- The spinal cord is the third most common site for metastasis after the lung and liver.
- Patients will often present with **pain** and, if **spinal cord compression** occurs, neurological deficit below the level of the metastasis.
- **MRI spine** is used for diagnosis of spinal metastases. Lesions are often multiple.
- Urgent dexamethasone should be administered followed by specialist advice regarding surgery or radiotherapy.

9.6 DISCITIS AND EPIDURAL ABSCESS

DEFINITION

- **Discitis** is infection or inflammation of the intervertebral disc; an **epidural abscess** represents infection within the epidural space:
  - Discitis usually occurs after haematogenous spread of infection from a distant site.
  - Epidural abscess usually results from direct introduction of bacteria into the epidural space (surgery, lumbar puncture, epidural anaesthesia) is more common.

CLINICAL FEATURES

- There is back pain with local inflammation and tenderness at the site of the lesion.
- Neurological deficit develops rapidly in epidural abscess (less commonly in discitis) and may produce myelopathy or radiculopathy.
- Systemic symptoms of infection such as fever and anorexia exist.

INVESTIGATIONS

- Elevated inflammatory markers.
- Blood cultures positive in a third of cases.
- Disc biopsy.
- Imaging, including an echocardiogram, to identify any deep source of infection if there is no history of instrumentation.
- **MRI spine** shows narrowing of the disc space and bone marrow oedema in discitis and will define an abscess if present.

MANAGEMENT

- Antibiotic therapy is given for at least 6 weeks.
- Emergency drainage of an abscess is usually required (especially if cord compression is present).
- Approximately 15% of patients are left with a permanent neurological deficit following discitis; this is more common with delayed diagnosis/treatment.

9.7 SUBACUTE COMBINED DEGENERATION (OF THE SPINAL CORD)

- Demyelination of the corticospinal tracts and dorsal columns of the spinal cord due to **vitamin B_{12} deficiency**.
    - Vitamin B_{12} deficiency impairs function of the enzymes methionine synthase and methymalonyl CoA mutase.
    - CNS implications of enzyme dysfunction are not well understood.
    - B_{12} deficiency also causes peripheral neuropathy.
- Vitamin B_{12} deficiency usually is due to either **poor dietary intake** (often alcoholism or a vegan diet) or **malabsorption** (pernicious anaemia, Crohn's disease, etc.).

CLINICAL FEATURES

- Typically, lower limbs are affected before upper limbs, with progressive motor and sensory deficit:
    - Early in the disease course, sensory symptoms predominate, with progressively ascending paraesthesia and sensory ataxia (due to a loss of proprioception).
    - Reflexes may be absent.
    - Later changes include a pyramidal pattern of weakness due to corticospinal tract damage (see Section 9.1, Spinal Cord Anatomy).

INVESTIGATIONS

- Macrocytic anaemia.
- Low serum vitamin B_{12} level.

Neurological zones

- Malabsorption screen (e.g. anti-tissue transglutaminase for coeliac disease).
  - **MRI spine** may show T2 hyperintensity, particularly in the thoracic dorsal columns.

MANAGEMENT

- Parenteral vitamin B_{12} (hydroxycobalamin) supplementation and treatment of any underlying malabsorptive syndrome are provided.
- Vitamin B_{12} replacement will prevent progression of the degeneration but rarely produces improvement.

9.8 MOTOR NEURON DISEASE

DEFINITION

- Motor neuron disease (MND) involves a heterogeneous group of progressive neurodegenerative disorders affecting upper and lower motor neurons.

PATHOPHYSIOLOGY

- Precise causes of selective neuronal death are not fully understood; possible mechanisms include oxidative stress, glutamate excitotoxicity, mitochondrial dysfunction, disordered axonal transport, protein aggregation and inflammation.

AETIOLOGY

- Usually idiopathic; approximately 10% are familial cases.
- Inheritance usually **autosomal dominant**; autosomal recessive and X-linked inheritance seen in some cases.
- Familial MND is genetically **heterogeneous**:
  - Until recently, the most common genetic variant was caused by mutations in the *SOD1* gene (accounts for 10–20% of familial MND).
  - Recently, a hexanucleotide expansion in the *C9ORF72* gene was discovered in up to 50% of familial MND; the disease mechanism in these cases remains unknown.

EPIDEMIOLOGY

- **Incidence**: approximately 1–2 per 100,000 population worldwide (sporadic MND).
- **Gender**: male/female ratio of approximately 1.6:1.
- **Age**: Onset is between 50 and 60 years, although rare juvenile-onset forms also exist.

CLINICAL FEATURES

- MND is subdivided into three main variants based on the pattern of **motor** symptoms:
    - **Amyotrophic lateral sclerosis (ALS)**: Loss of motor neurons in the motor cortex and anterior horn of spinal cord produces **upper and lower motor neuron** features.
    - **Primary lateral sclerosis (PLS)** (1–3%): Includes **purely upper motor neuron** features and pseudobulbar palsy. Often progresses to ALS.
    - **Progressive muscular atrophy (PMA)** (10%): Loss of motor neurons in the anterior horn of the spinal cord causes a **purely lower motor neuron** syndrome. It often starts asymmetrically, affecting distal muscle groups before spreading proximally.
- There is **no sensory involvement**; the presence of mixed upper and lower motor neuron symptoms in the absence of sensory signs is almost **diagnostic** for MND.
- Notably, the **extraocular** muscles and **bladder** function are largely spared in the disease process.
- A proportion of patients with MND suffer extramotor disease, usually **frontotemporal dementia**.

INVESTIGATIONS

- There is no definitive test for MND, and diagnosis relies largely on clinical assessment.
- **Electromyography (EMG)**: shows fibrillation and fasciculation potential activity.
- **Nerve conduction studies**: show normal sensory conduction and mainly normal motor conduction.
- Exclude alternate causes, for example, by MRI of brain and spinal cord, CSF analysis and muscle biopsy.

MANAGEMENT

- Currently, MND is **incurable**; **counselling** is important for the patient and family.
- **Riluzole** (glutamate release inhibitor) slows disease progression and increases survival by 3–4 months.
- **MDT approach** is required, involving neurologist, specialist nurse, physiotherapist, occupational therapist, dietician, speech therapist, social worker and GP.
- **Symptomatic treatment**:
    - **dysphagia**: blended food, nutritional supplements, gastrostomy;
    - **drooling of saliva**: hyoscine patch, atropine, amitriptyline or botulinum toxin injection into salivary glands;
    - **dysarthria**: electronic communication device;

Neurological zones

- **muscle weakness**: physiotherapy, walking aids;
- **spasticity**: baclofen, dantrolene, physiotherapy;
- **constipation**: assess fibre intake, bulk-forming or osmotic laxatives, glycerol suppositories;
- **depression/emotional lability**: tricyclic agents or selective serotonin reuptake inhibitors;
- **urinary disturbance**: amitriptyline, oxybutinin or detrusitol;
- **dyspnoea**: non-invasive intermittent ventilation (NIV) is effective for relieving nocturnal hypoventilation, improving quality of life and extending survival.

PROGNOSIS

- The clinical course of MND is highly variable; death from respiratory failure typically occurs within 2–5 years from onset of symptoms.

MICRO-case

Vertebral disc prolapse

A 50-year-old builder presents to the GP with back pain, which is preventing him from working. It started 5 days ago when he was lifting some bricks, and he felt his back 'go'. Since then, he has had pain in the back, radiating to the left buttock and down the back of the leg. He has tried simple analgesia, but it has made no difference. Lifting heavy objects and sitting for long periods of time exacerbate the symptoms. His bowel and bladder function is normal. He has had no previous injuries to his back and is normally fit and well.

On examination, he has no pain on palpation of the spine but does experience pain on palpation of the left buttock. He has no weakness, but his movement is significantly limited by pain, which radiates from his buttock to his foot. There is no altered sensation, and his reflexes are normal. Straight leg raise testing is positive.

The diagnosis of sciatica is made. The patient is encouraged to mobilise, given simple exercises to complete, and prescribed paracetamol and diclofenac to help with the pain. He is asked to make a further appointment in 6 weeks for a review and is given a sick note to excuse him from work for this time period. He is told that if his symptoms worsen or he experiences problems with his bowel or bladder habits, it is important to seek medical attention immediately.

Summary points

- Back pain is a very common presenting complaint, especially in patients with manual jobs.

continued…

continued...

- It is vital to exclude cord compression in these patients. If there is no neurological deficit, then conservative management is appropriate.
- Patients with sciatica should remain as active as possible; swimming, walking and gentle stretching can be very beneficial.
- Use a safety net in all patients with back pain; make an appointment for a review and ensure they know to seek medical attention if symptoms worsen or if signs of cord compression develop.

10 Peripheral nervous system

10.1 ANATOMY OF THE PERIPHERAL NERVOUS SYSTEM

- The peripheral nervous system is comprised of somatic (motor and sensory) and autonomic (motor, sensory and secretomotor) components.
- It connects the central nervous system (CNS) (brain and spinal cord) to the rest of the body and is made up of:
  - cranial nerves – from brainstem nuclei;
  - peripheral nerves – formed from spinal nerves.
- In the cervical and lumbosacral regions, spinal roots are formed into peripheral nerves via **plexi**.
  - The **cervical plexus** is formed from spinal roots C1–C4 and supplies muscles and skin of the posterior head and neck. It is located deep to the sternocleidomastoid muscle.
  - The **brachial plexus**, formed from roots C5–T1, supplies muscles and skin of the upper limb and is located in the neck, axilla and proximal upper limb (see **Fig. 10.1**).
  - The **lumbosacral plexus** is a combination of two joined plexi (lumbar and sacral). It is formed from spinal roots T12–L4 (lumbar plexus) and L4–S5 (sacral plexus) and supplies the lower limb and pelvis (see **Fig. 10.2**).

IMPORTANT PERIPHERAL NERVES

- **Ulnar nerve**: supplies all of the small muscles of the hand except those supplied by the **median nerve**. Also supplies the flexor carpi ulnaris and half of the flexor digitorum profundus in the forearm.
- **Median nerve**: supplies all of the forearm flexors (except those supplied by the ulnar nerve); also supplies the lateral two **l**umbricals, **o**pponens pollicis, **a**bductor pollicis brevis and **f**lexor pollicis brevis (**LOAF**) in the hand.
- **Radial nerve**: supplies the forearm extensors.
- See **Fig. 10.3**.
- **Common peroneal nerve**: supplies muscles responsible for ankle dorsiflexion and foot eversion (see **Fig. 10.4**).

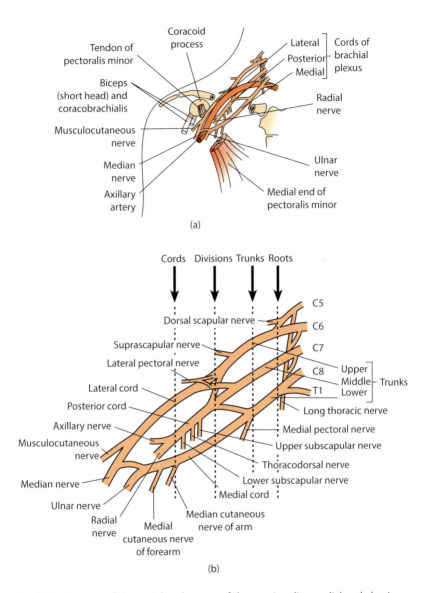

(a)

(b)

Fig. 10.1 Diagram of the peripheral nerves of the arm (median, radial and ulnar) illustrating their origin as spinal root and their formation via the brachial plexus.

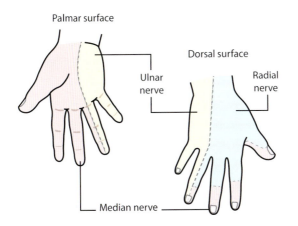

Fig. 10.2 Illustration of the area of skin supplied by each of the median, radial and ulnar nerves.

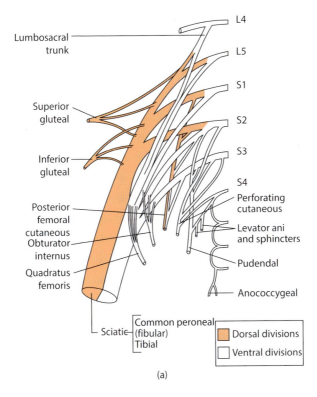

(a)

Fig. 10.3 Diagram of the peripheral nerves of the leg illustrating (a) their origin as spinal root.

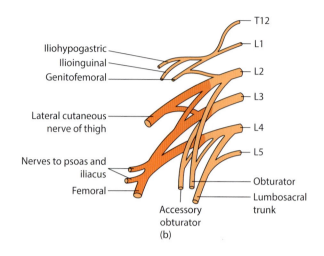

Fig. 10.3 (*Continued*) Diagram of the peripheral nerves of the leg illustrating (b) their formation via the lumbosacral plexus.

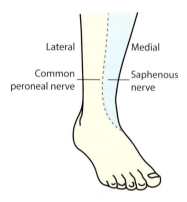

Fig. 10.4 Illustration of the area of skin supplied by the common peroneal and saphenous vein nerve.

10.2 ENTRAPMENT NEUROPATHIES

CARPAL TUNNEL SYNDROME

DEFINITION

- Compression of the **median nerve** as it passes through the carpal tunnel at the wrist, producing motor and sensory dysfunction.

PATHOPHYSIOLOGY

- The carpal tunnel contains the tendons of the forearm flexor muscles as well as the median nerve and is roofed over by the relatively rigid flexor retinaculum.

- Any reduction of space within the carpal tunnel leaves the median nerve vulnerable to compression.

AETIOLOGY

The following are conditions associated with a reduction of volume in the carpal tunnel:
- pregnancy;
- obesity;
- hypothyroidism;
- rheumatoid arthritis;
- acromegaly.

CLINICAL FEATURES

- **Paraesthesia**:
    - This occurs over the thumb, index and middle fingers and the radial half of the ring finger.
    - Sensation over the palm and thenar eminence is unaffected as the palmar cutaneous branch of the median nerve leaves the nerve proximal to the wrist and does not pass through the carpal tunnel.
    - It is worse at night due to prolonged flexion and fluid retention.
- Weakness and wasting of the muscles of the thenar eminence occur.
- Tinel's and Phalen's signs may be positive, but they are unreliable signs.

MICRO-print

Both Tinel's and Phalen's signs use manoeuvres to reproduce carpal tunnel syndrome symptoms.

- **Tinel's sign**: tapping over the flexor retinaculum.
- **Phalen's sign**: holding the wrist in fixed flexion for a prolonged period.

INVESTIGATIONS

- Nerve conduction studies (NCS) and electromyography (EMG).

MANAGEMENT

- Initially conservative treatment:
    - education;
    - nocturnal splinting; to keep the wrist in extension.
- Steroid injection into the carpal tunnel.
- Surgical release of the flexor retinaculum for patients with motor symptoms.

Neurological zones

ULNAR NERVE PALSY

- The ulnar nerve is very superficial at several points along its course; it is thus vulnerable to damage due to external compression:
  - Usually occurs in the cubital tunnel at the elbow, but other vulnerable areas include Guyon's canal in the wrist.
- Often, this palsy is a result of fracture or dislocation of the elbow or compression from leaning on the elbow on a hard surface for a prolonged period.

CLINICAL FEATURES

- Vary according to the site of compression. More proximal compression results in less-severe deformity due to paralysis of forearm flexors (ulnar paradox).
  - **Injury at the wrist:**
    - sensory loss over the little finger;
    - weakness of all ulnar-innervated muscles in the hand but not the forearm flexors; the unopposed action of the long flexors on the two medial fingers means they cannot be extended – the 'ulnar claw' (more apparent on attempting to extend the fingers).
  - **Injury at the elbow:**
    - sensory loss over the dorsal aspect of the hand, the ring, little and ulnar half of the middle finger;
    - weakness and wasting of most of the small muscles of the hand, including the hypothenar eminence, and the long flexors of the ring and little fingers;
    - paralysis of the interossei and medial two lumbricals result in claw hand deformity.

MANAGEMENT

- Transient compression at the elbow may resolve spontaneously; splinting of the elbow in extension can aid recovery.
- Surgical decompression of cubital tunnel may be required.

MICRO-print

Common peroneal nerve palsy

- The common peroneal nerve runs superficially around the neck of the **fibula**. It is vulnerable to compression or damage in fractures of the fibula.
- Damage to the nerve will produce altered sensation over the dorsum of the foot and lateral calf. Patients also develop weakness of dorsiflexion (i.e. foot drop) and eversion at the ankle.
- Many common peroneal nerve palsies respond to conservative management. Fracture of the fibula may require surgical intervention.

continued...

continued...

Radial nerve palsy ('Saturday Night' palsy)

- Compression of the radial nerve as it leaves the posterior cord of the brachial plexus or in the radial groove over the lateral humerus.
- May result in prominent wrist drop due to paralysis of the forearm extensor muscles and altered sensation in a small area over the dorsum of the wrist.
- Many radial nerve palsies will respond to conservative management.

Median nerve palsy (proximal)

- Usually, proximal median nerve palsy is due to trauma to the arm or forearm or damage to the nerve as it leaves the brachial plexus.
- A very proximal injury to the nerve will produce weakness of wrist flexion (some flexion preserved due to ulnar innervation of some flexor muscles) and of flexion of the two lateral fingers – more apparent when trying to make a fist.
- The intrinsic hand muscles supplied by the median nerve will also be weakened, and sensory loss will occur in the pattern described previously (including loss of palmar sensation).

MICRO-print
Mononeuritis multiplex

- Asymmetrical asynchronous palsy of a number of peripheral nerves, often due to inflammation.
- Causes include:
  - diabetes mellitus;
  - infiltrative: amyloidosis;
  - inflammatory: vasculitis and sarcoidosis;
  - infective: Lyme disease, leprosy and HIV;
  - malignant: carcinomatosis or paraneoplastic.
- Aside from investigations for these causes, a positron emission tomographic (PET) scan may be useful for identifying malignancy or vasculitis.

10.3 PLEXOPATHIES

- Plexopathies are lesions affecting one of the nervous plexuses; the brachial plexus is most commonly affected.

CLINICAL FEATURES

- Lesions of the **brachial plexus** result in unilateral neurological deficit affecting both motor and sensory function in the upper limb.

- Lesions of the **lumbosacral plexus** produce unilateral weakness and sensory loss of the affected lower limb.
- Causes of plexopathy include:
  - malignant infiltration of a plexus;
  - diabetes;
  - post-radiotherapy;
  - compression: the lumbar plexus is contained within the psoas muscle; a psoas haematoma may result in compression.
- In addition to these causes, brachial plexopathy may result from:
  - neuralgic amyotrophy – idiopathic inflammation;
  - trauma to the proximal arm/axilla;
  - Klumpke's paralysis (T1 nerve root avulsion): results from forceful arm abduction;
  - Erb's palsy (C5–C6 nerve root avulsion): due to forceful traction of the head, often during an instrumental delivery;
  - thoracic outlet syndrome.
- MRI of the plexus is used to look for a structural lesion; NCS and EMG are also helpful.

10.4 POLYNEUROPATHIES

OVERVIEW

DEFINITION

- Dysfunction of peripheral nerves distal to a plexus, often a result of a widespread disease process.

CLINICAL FEATURES

- Vary according to the cause, but some common features are useful in distinguishing polyneuropathy from more proximal dysfunction:
  - Distal distribution of symptoms; legs are usually affected before arms.
  - Symptoms may be sensory (paraesthesia and pain), motor (distal weakness) or both.
    - Weakness is in a lower motor neuron disease pattern.
- Sensory change may vary according to the type of fibre affected:
  - **Large myelinated fibres**: numbness, paraesthesia and sensory ataxia. Romberg's test is positive.
  - **Small myelinated** and **non-myelinated fibres**: numbness or a painful sensation classically described as 'burning'. Normally painless stimuli may become painful or unpleasant (**allodynia**).
- Autonomic dysfunction is a feature of some polyneuropathies.

 AETIOLOGY

- **Acquired axonal polyneuropathies**:
  - Many cases are idiopathic.
  - Typically, these are slowly progressive and predominantly sensory.
  - Causes include diabetes mellitus, alcohol and metabolic causes such as liver or renal failure, porphyria and vitamin B_{12} deficiency.
- **Acquired demyelinating polyneuropathies**:
  - typically inflammatory;
  - include Guillain–Barré syndrome and chronic inflammatory demyelinating polyneuropathy (CIDP).
- **Infections** (e.g. Lyme disease).
- **Toxins**: alcohol, drugs (phenytoin, isoniazid, anti-retrovirals).
- **Infiltrative** or **vasculitic**: amyloidosis, sarcoidosis.
- **Malignancy**: usually related to a paraneoplastic syndrome – mixed motor and sensory loss.
- **Inherited**: hereditary motor and sensory neuropathy (HMSN; Charcot–Marie–Tooth disease).

MICRO-print

Pattern of neurological symptoms in peripheral neuropathies

PREDOMINANT MOTOR	MIXED MOTOR AND SENSORY	PREDOMINANT SENSORY
Guillain–Barré syndrome	HMSN	Diabetes
CIDP	Amyloidosis	Vitamin B_{12} deficiency
Acute porphyria	Alcohol	Uraemia

GUILLAIN–BARRÉ SYNDROME (GBS)

DEFINITION

- An acute inflammatory demyelinating polyradiculoneuropathy (AIDP).
- The axonal variant (acute motor axonal neuropathy, AMAN) carries a worse prognosis and is associated with *Campylobacter jejuni*.

AETIOLOGY

- Approximately 75% of cases follow an infective illness up to 6 weeks earlier:
  - non-specific lower respiratory tract infection;
  - 25% of cases associated with **_Campylobacter jejuni_** gastroenteritis.

Neurological zones

Pathophysiology

- Triggered by an immune cross-reactivity; antibodies directed at the infectious organism also target components of the peripheral nerves.
- Affects roots as well as peripheral nerve.
- Classically described as ascending paralysis but can cause proximal or a pseudopyramidal pattern of weakness.

Epidemiology

- **Incidence**: approximately 2 per 100,000 population per year.
- **Gender**: more common in males than females.
- **Age**: more common in middle age.

Clinical features

- Onset over hours–days with peak in symptom severity within 4 weeks.
- Ascending weakness; proximal weakness may be prominent. Respiratory muscle involvement may necessitate ventilation.
- Sensory loss is variable.
- Neurological deficit may be preceded by back pain.

Investigations

- **Cerebrospinal fluid (CSF) examination**: typically elevated protein with a normal white cell count. A slight lymphocytosis can occur (<50 cells/μl).
- **NCS/EMG**: Classically a proximal demyelination of motor nerves is demonstrated. A conduction block may be present.
- **Respiratory function**: A decline in forced vital capacity (FVC) indicating respiratory muscle weakness will require ventilatory support.

Management

- **Intravenous immunoglobulin**: first-line management for Guillain-Barré syndrome.
- **Plasmapheresis**:
  - This is second-line treatment if no improvement following intravenous immunoglobulin.
  - The aim of this therapy is to remove autoantibodies from the blood.
- Development of respiratory muscle weakness should precipitate transfer to a high-dependency area.
- Artificial ventilation may be necessary to maintain respiration until muscle weakness has improved.

Prognosis

- Most patients make a full recovery; about 20% are left with mild residual weakness or sensory loss.

Neurological zones

- Mortality is about 5% due to respiratory failure, thromboembolic events or secondary infection.

> **MICRO-print**
>
> **Chronic inflammatory demyelinating polyradiculoneuropathy**
>
> - CIDP is an inflammatory polyneuropathy with demyelination of peripheral nerves.
> - Symptoms in CIDP usually present over a period of weeks–months. In addition, CIDP produces relapses.
> - Investigation is as for Guillain–Barré syndrome. EMG/NCS are often diagnostic.
> - **Immunosuppression** with corticosteroids is helpful in CIDP. Intravenous immunoglobulin and plasmapheresis alongside corticosteroids may be helpful for acute relapses.
> - The prognosis in CIDP is variable, but many patients are left with some residual neurological deficit between relapses.

DIABETIC POLYNEUROPATHY

PATHOPHYSIOLOGY

- Long-term hyperglycaemia produces small nerve fibre damage.
- The exact mechanism is unknown, but accumulation of sorbitol in peripheral nerves and microvascular dysfunction are implicated.

EPIDEMIOLOGY

- **Prevalance**: About 15% of diabetics have significant peripheral neuropathy (increases with disease duration). This usually develops about 10 years after the development of diabetes.
- **Gender**: Develops earlier in males than females.
- More common with increasing duration of disease and poor glycaemic control.

CLINICAL FEATURES

- Predominantly a sensory neuropathy, but all modalities may be affected, with involvement of both small and large fibres.
- **Autonomic dysfunction**: postural hypotension, erectile dysfunction.
- Proximal motor neuropathy (diabetic amyotrophy):
  - asymmetrical weakness and wasting of proximal leg muscles with associated pain;
  - occasionally precipitated by rapid improvement of glycaemic control.

INVESTIGATION

- Monitoring of glycaemic control and HbA1c.
- NCS/EMG may be useful.

Management

- **Improvement of glycaemic control**: Slows progression but does not reverse nerve damage.
- **Analgesia**: Duloxetine is the first-line treatment for painful diabetic polyneuropathy.
- **Prevention of neuropathic ulceration**: Education on foot care and referral to a podiatrist.
- Autonomic dysfunction regulation:
    - **fludrocortisone** for postural hypotension;
    - **sildenafil** for erectile dysfunction.

HEREDITARY MOTOR AND SENSORY NEUROPATHY (CHARCOT–MARIE–TOOTH DISEASE)

- A collection of heterogeneous, inherited, slowly progressive polyneuropathies with both motor and sensory dysfunction.
- Mutations within myelin or Schwann's cells responsible for nerve myelination.
- Prevalence is 1 per 2500 population; most common inherited neuromuscular disorder.
- Affects males and females equally.
- Can be very slowly progressive but may become clinically evident before the age of 20 years.

Clinical features

- Motor symptoms tend to predominate.
- **Pes cavus**: fixed plantar flexion of the foot that is often combined with inversion of the hindfoot.
- Sensation may be normal, or patients may experience some numbness, but painful dysathesia is very uncommon.
- In HMSN type I, there is hypertrophy of the nerves.

Investigation

- NCS/EMG; genetic testing may be diagnostic.

Management

- There is no disease-modifying therapy for HMSN.
- Symptomatic treatment includes:
    - reducing discomfort associated with foot deformities;
    - physiotherapy and the provision of orthoses;
    - corrective orthopaedic surgery for refractive cases.
- Genetic counselling should be provided to patients and their families.

PROGNOSIS

- Life expectancy in HMSN is not altered except in the most severe cases.

10.5 HORNER'S SYNDROME

DEFINITION

- A combination of ptosis and miosis with or without reduced sweating over the face on the side of the affected eye.

PATHOPHYSIOLOGY

- Pathology within the ipsilateral sympathetic outflow between the cervical spinal cord and the effector organs in the eye.

AETIOLOGY

- Horner's syndrome may result from pathology affecting the first-, second- or third-order neuron of the sympathetic supply to the eye/face.
- **First-order neuron**: pathology of the cervical spinal cord.
- **Second-order preganglionic neuron** (between the spinal cord and the sympathetic chain):
    - **malignancy**: especially tumour in the apex of the lung that invades the sympathetic outflow (Pancoast's tumour);
    - cervical rib;
    - cervical lymphadenopathy.
- **Third-order postganglionic neuron**:
    - Divergence of the sympathetic supply to the eye and face occurs at the sympathetic ganglion; absence of anhydrosis is indicative of a third-order nerve lesion. Causes include:
        - internal carotid artery dissection;
        - carotid body tumour;
        - cluster headaches;
        - caroto-cavernous sinus fistula.

INVESTIGATION

- **Chest X-ray**: identify an apical lung tumour.
- MRI head and neck.
- **Apraclonidine**:
    - an α-2 and α-1 adrenergic receptor agonist;
    - topical administration produces pupillary dilation in Horner syndrome due to loss of sympathetic innervation and upregulation of α-1 receptors.

MANAGEMENT

- Dependent on the cause.

Neurological zones

MICRO-case

Guillain–Barré syndrome

A 48-year-old gentleman presented to the emergency department with a 3-day history of leg weakness. He initially noticed that he was beginning to trip over his own feet, and then walking became increasingly difficult. That day, he had noticed that his hands were weaker than usual as he was unable to remove the lid from a jar of coffee. He denied any change in sensation or pain in his limbs, and, on further questioning, reported no other neurological deficit. He had no history of any similar previous episodes of weakness or any other neurological deficit. Two weeks previously, he saw his general practitioner (GP) for an acute diarrhoeal illness that developed after attending a friend's barbecue. He had noticed some blood in his stools and had several episodes of fever, but his bowel habit has now returned to normal without any treatment. On examination, the power in his lower limbs was reduced throughout, with slightly reduced tone. His reflexes were diminished, with mute plantars. There was moderate impairment of light touch and vibration sense to the level of the knees bilaterally. In the arms, he had bilateral weakness with markedly reduced grip strength and normal tone. Reflexes were hard to elicit. Sensation appeared intact. Cranial nerve examination was entirely normal, as was his FVC.

A lumbar puncture was performed and CSF examination revealed a white cell count of 4 cells/µl (100% lymphocytes), a glucose concentration of 3.2 mmol/l (serum concentration 5.4 mmol/L) and a protein concentration of 1.4 g/L. EMG/NCS were consistent with a demyelinating polyneuropathy.

A diagnosis of Guillain–Barré syndrome was made, and he was commenced on intravenous immunoglobulin. His weakness progressed for several days after admission, but 3 weeks after the onset of his symptoms his deficit began to improve. During his admission, his FVC was monitored several times a day. Over the next month, he made a full recovery with the help of physiotherapy input.

Summary points

- EMG and NCS are useful for investigation for disorders of the peripheral nervous system.
- It is important to investigate for other common causes of peripheral neuropathy to avoid misdiagnosis.
- Guillain–Barré is a potentially dangerous condition, and close monitoring for respiratory muscle weakness is essential.

Neurological zones

11 Neuromuscular junction and muscle

11.1 ANATOMY AND PHYSIOLOGY

- See **Fig. 11.1**.
- The neuromuscular junction (NMJ) allows motor neurons to stimulate contraction of muscles:
  - The depolarizing action potential arriving at the presynaptic terminal opens voltage-gated calcium channels, stimulating exocytosis of acetylcholine into the synaptic cleft.
  - The acetylcholine diffuses across the cleft to act on the post-synaptic receptors.
  - The acetylcholine receptors (AChRs) are ligand-gated ion channels; when stimulated, they open to allow sodium ion influx down a concentration gradient to cause a local depolarization, which stimulates muscle contraction.
- Acetylcholine esterase breaks down acetylcholine in the synaptic cleft. This is one mechanism for limiting the duration of a muscle contraction in response to a nerve signal.
- Disorders of the NMJ are characterized by weakness, typically of the larger proximal muscles, due to impaired transmission across the NMJ.

11.2 MYASTHENIA GRAVIS

DEFINITION

- Myasthenia gravis (MG) is an autoimmune disease of the NMJ, producing fatigable muscle weakness.
- **Post-synaptic disorder**.

AETIOLOGY

- Autoimmune, antibody-mediated disease caused by:
  - antibodies to post-synaptic acetylcholine receptors (anti-AChRs) – 80% of cases;
  - antibodies to muscle-specific tyrosine kinase (MuSK).
- Seronegative disease can occur with no detectable antibodies.
- Treatment with penicillamine (e.g. in rheumatoid arthritis) can produce a transient myasthenic syndrome – anti-AChR present.

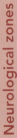

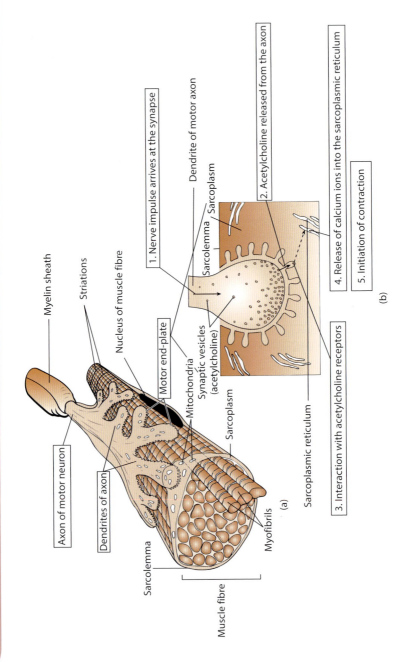

Myelin sheath

Striations

Nucleus of muscle fibre

1. Nerve impulse arrives at the synapse

Dendrite of motor axon

Sarcoplasm

Sarcolemma

2. Acetylcholine released from the axon

4. Release of calcium ions into the sarcoplasmic reticulum

5. Initiation of contraction

Motor end-plate

Mitochondria

Synaptic vesicles (acetylcholine)

Sarcoplasm

3. Interaction with acetylcholine receptors

Sarcoplasmic reticulum

Axon of motor neuron

Dendrites of axon

Sarcolemma

Muscle fibre

Myofibrils

(a)

(b)

Fig. 11.1 Diagram of neuromuscular junction: (a) a motor unit and (b) ultrastructure of the neuromuscular synapse.

PATHOPHYSIOLOGY

- **Anti-AChR positive**:
  - Anti-AChR antibodies are produced by plasma cells and bind to post-synaptic receptors.
  - They cause damage or destruction of post-synaptic receptors.
  - Fewer functioning post-synaptic receptors reduce the influx of sodium ions in response to a synaptic impulse, resulting in weakness.
  - Particularly affects repeated synaptic impulses where receptors have been temporarily used up by previous contractions.
- **Anti-MuSK positive**:
  - MuSK is important for AChR clustering at the postsynaptic membrane.
- The thymus is implicated in pathogenesis due to its role in plasma cell maturation. Up to 75% have an abnormality of the thymus (e.g. hyperplasia or thymoma).

EPIDEMIOLOGY

- **Gender**: females more than males (2:1).
- **Age**: bimodal peak age of incidence at 30 years and 50–70 years.

CLINICAL FEATURES

- **Weakness**:
  - worsens with exercise (fatigability);
  - not confined to a nerve or nerve root distribution;
  - reflex present but also fatigable;
  - common patterns:
    - proximal limb weakness;
    - ophthalmoplegia: diplopia and ptosis;
    - bulbar weakness: dysphagia and dysarthria.
- Onset of symptoms usually over several weeks/months; symptoms may be precipitated by an intercurrent illness.
- Can present with a myasthenic crisis (see the following MICRO-facts).

MICRO-facts

Myasthenic crisis may occur in patients with known MG or may be the first presentation. May be difficult to distinguish from cholinergic crisis, which is due to overmedication with anti-cholinesterase inhibitor.

A typical myasthenic crisis involves generalised worsening weakness, including breathlessness and bulbar weakness, which can lead to respiratory failure and aspiration respectively. *continued...*

continued...

Neurological zones

> **continued...**
>
> **Management**
> - Monitor respiratory function; may require intubation and ventilation.
> - Plasmapheresis or intravenous immunoglobulin.
> - Stop any acetylcholinesterase inhibitor treatment temporarily.

INVESTIGATIONS

- **Diagnostic tests**:
  - **Serology**: autoantibodies usually detectable in the serum of symptomatic patients (90% of patients with generalised symptoms; 50% of patients with only ocular symptoms).
  - **Neurophysiological studies**: repetitive motor nerve stimulation shows a decreasing muscle response.
  - If serology and NCS non-diagnostic, consider Tensilon® (edrophonium) test:
    - An intravenous anticholinesterase agent (edrophonium) is administered, first as a test dose of 2 mg, then a further 8 mg.
    - In myasthenia gravis, a marked improvement in muscle power is seen within 5 minutes of edrophonium administration.
    - Resuscitation facilities, including **atropine**, must be on hand as the cholinergic effects of edrophonium may include severe bradycardia.
- **Other tests**:
  - **Imaging**: Chest X-ray or computed tomography (CT) of the thorax may identify thymic hyperplasia or a thymoma.
  - **Pulmonary function testing**: Spirometry to assess for respiratory muscle weakness is extremely important. During a relapse, monitoring of the forced vital capacity (FVC) to allow early intervention is crucial.

MANAGEMENT

- **Acetylcholinesterase inhibitors** (e.g. pyridostigmine, neostigmine):
  - inhibit the action of cholinesterases at the NMJ and therefore increase the availability of acetylcholine;
  - produce symptomatic relief but have no effect on the progressive destruction of AChRs;
  - over-medication can produce a cholinergic crisis (atropine treatment required).
- **Immunosuppression**: usually with corticosteroids. Azathioprine is frequently used as a steroid-sparing agent.
- **Immunoglobulins/plasmapheresis**: used in patients who are rapidly deteriorating or in myasthenic crisis.
- **Thymectomy**: should be performed in patients with a thymoma.
- Ventilatory support may be required with severe respiratory muscle weakness.

PROGNOSIS

- With treatment, patients have a normal life expectancy.
- Respiratory failure, often complicated by aspiration pneumonia, is a life-threatening complication of MG.

11.3 LAMBERT–EATON MYASTHENIC SYNDROME

DEFINITION

- Lambert–Eaton myasthenic syndrome (LEMS) is a **presynaptic** neuromuscular disorder with weakness that improves with exercise.

AETIOLOGY

- Usually occurs as a paraneoplastic syndrome (particularly with small-cell lung cancer).
- Can occur as an autoimmune condition.

PATHOPHYSIOLOGY

- Release of acetylcholine from nerve endings is reduced, causing impaired impulse transmission across the NMJ.
- Antibodies to **presynaptic voltage-gated calcium channels** are found in 90% of patients.
  - Presynaptic influx of calcium is important in initiating exocytosis of neurotransmitter.

CLINICAL FEATURES

- **Proximal muscle weakness** – improves briefly with vigorous exercise.
  - Ocular, bulbar and respiratory muscles usually only mildly affected.
  - Reduced reflexes are present, which return/increase with muscle exertion.
- **Autonomic dysfunction** can occur (e.g. dry mouth, gastroparesis, constipation, erectile dysfunction).

DIAGNOSIS

- **Serology**: Antibodies to voltage-gated calcium channels are detected in around 90% of patients (specific to LEMS).
- **Neurophysiological studies**: Repetitive motor nerve stimulation shows an increasing muscle response.
- Further investigations can be made for possible malignancy (e.g. CT scanning).

MANAGEMENT

- **Immunosuppression**:
  - Immunosuppression is less effective than in other autoimmune diseases, including myasthenia gravis.
  - Corticosteroids and azathioprine used earlier in the course of LEMS than in MG.

Neurological zones

- Intravenous immunoglobulin and plasmapheresis may be used in acute severe weakness.
- **Other treatments**:
  - Acetylcholinesterase inhibitors (e.g. pyridostigmine) produce symptomatic improvement.
  - 3,4-Diaminopyridine (3,4-DAP) increases the release of acetylcholine and improves weakness.
  - Treatment of any underlying malignancy.

Prognosis

- Long-term outcome is largely dependent on the presence of an underlying malignancy.
- Diagnosis of LEMS can lead to early detection of small-cell lung cancer and thus improve prognosis.
- If no malignancy is detected 2 years after onset of symptoms, then the disease is likely to be autoimmune; prognosis then is usually good because of relative sparing of respiratory and bulbar muscles.

11.4 BOTULISM

- Toxin produced by *Clostridium botulinum* bacterium inhibits the release of acetylcholine at the NMJ (**presynaptic disorder**) and in terminal synapses of the parasympathetic nervous system.
- Infection occurs after ingestion of contaminated foods (commonly canned food) or from a contaminated wound.
- Incidence of wound botulism is increasing related to injection of heroin directly into skin and muscle ('skin-popping').

Clinical features

- Symptoms of food-borne botulism and wound botulism are similar except that the incubation period is shorter in food contamination (~1 day) compared to wound contamination (~10 days).
- A higher inoculating dose of toxin will produce symptoms more rapidly.
- **Weakness**:
  - Progressive, symmetrical descending weakness occurs.
  - Cranial nerve symptoms (e.g. diplopia, ptosis, dysarthria, dysphagia) occur early, followed by respiratory and limb weakness.
- Anticholinergic symptoms
  - Dilated pupils, dry mouth, constipation, urinary retention and postural hypotension.
- Gastrointestinal symptoms are more prominent in food botulism.

Investigations

- Diagnosis is largely clinical.

- Serology may detect botulinum toxin in blood.
- Neurophysiological studies show increasing response to stimulation.

MANAGEMENT

- Respiratory depression can occur quickly, so patients require close monitoring of respiratory function, including FVC. Early ventilation may be required.
- **Antitoxin** should be given once the clinical diagnosis is made. This will not reverse paralysis but prevents progression.
- Wound botulism requires thorough debridement of the wound site; antibiotics may be used.
- Botulism is a notifiable disease.

PROGNOSIS

- With effective supportive care, botulism should have no long-term sequelae.

MICRO-case
Myasthenia gravis

A 68-year-old woman visits her general practitioner (GP) with a 4-week history of double vision, which is better in the morning and becomes worse throughout the day. She thinks her speech becomes slurred towards the end of the day; she has trouble getting out of her chair in the evenings and becomes breathless climbing the stairs. She has no pain or rashes and is otherwise well. She mentions that people have commented that her eyelids look 'droopy'. She denies any weight loss or chest symptoms.

On examination, she has bilateral ptosis, but pupils are normal. She begins to slur her words when asked to count to a hundred. She reports diplopia on testing, and she has a complex ophthalmoplegia. She has 4+/5 proximal weakness, normal reflexes, no muscle tenderness or sensory loss. Her FVC is 1.2.

Her ptosis and limb weakness improve markedly but transiently on administration of intravenous edrophonium, and a diagnosis of MG is made. Immunology results 1 month later reveal positive anti-AChR antibodies.

Summary points
- Weakness in MG affects the ocular, facial and proximal limb muscles.
- Ocular involvement, especially complex ophthalmoplegia (weakness of both eyes not explained by a single cranial nerve lesion), is very suggestive of MG.
- Respiratory muscle involvement should be excluded in all cases with regular FVC monitoring, and patients may require ventilation and management in an intensive care unit.

11.5 INFLAMMATORY MYOPATHY

DEFINITIONS

- Polymyositis and dermatomyositis are autoimmune inflammatory conditions affecting skeletal muscle.
- Dermatomyositis is associated with characteristic dermatological symptoms.

EPIDEMIOLOGY

- **Incidence**: approximately 1 per 200,000 population per year.
- **Gender**: more common in women (2:1).

AETIOLOGY

- Polymyositis and dermatomyositis are both autoimmune connective tissue disorders. There is a strong association with other similar conditions, such as rheumatoid arthritis, systemic lupus erythematosus (SLE) and Sjögren's syndrome.

PATHOPHYSIOLOGY

- **Polymyositis**: Muscle necrosis occurs when cytotoxic T cells attack muscle fibres.
- **Dermatomyositis**: Inflammatory changes lead to damage of muscle capillaries, causing ischaemia.

CLINICAL FEATURES

- **Polymyositis**:
  - Weakness of proximal limb and girdle muscles occurs.
  - Muscle wasting can develop.
  - Ocular muscles are spared.
  - Distal muscles (e.g. hand muscles) are affected only very late in disease process.
  - Pain is present in weak muscles (occurs in one-third of patients).
  - Muscle weakness varies in severity over time.
  - Involvement of respiratory and bulbar muscles can cause dyspnoea and dysphagia.
- **Dermatomyositis**:
  - Muscle weakness is similar to polymyositis.
  - Symptoms associated with connective tissue disease may occur, including fever, weight loss, Raynaud's syndrome and pulmonary fibrosis.
  - Heliotrope rash: characteristic purple rash affecting the upper eyelids and around the eyes.
  - Gottron's papules: erythematous rash affecting extensor surfaces of joints.
- Dermatomyositis is often paraneoplastic. Between 10% and 20% of patients with dermatomyositis have an underlying malignancy; this percentage is higher in patients over 50 years old.

INVESTIGATIONS

- **Blood tests**:
  - Serum creatinine phosphokinase (CPK) is elevated (up to 50 times the upper limit of normal); however, a normal CPK does not exclude the diagnosis.
  - Inflammatory markers, including C-reactive protein and erythrocyte sedimentation rate, are usually raised.
- **Serology**:
  - Anti-nuclear antibody is positive in approximately 60%.
  - Around 20% of patients will have anti-Jo-1 autoantibodies. These are associated with Raynaud's syndrome, pulmonary fibrosis and poor response to treatment.
- **Neurophysiological studies**: Electromyography shows a myopathic picture (short, spiky polyphasic action potentials).
- **Histology**:
  - Muscle biopsy is required for definitive diagnosis.
  - Biopsy shows muscle fibre atrophy and inflammatory changes; findings vary according to exact pathology.
- Elderly patients with dermatomyositis should be investigated (e.g. via mammogram, colonoscopy, chest X-ray) for an underlying malignancy.

MANAGEMENT

- **Corticosteroids**: Dose should be titrated to CPK levels. High doses may be necessary acutely.
- **Steroid-sparing agents**: Drugs such as mycophenolate and cyclophosphamide can be used alone or in conjunction with corticosteroids.
- **Monoclonal antibody therapy**: Rituximab (anti-CD20) has been shown to be beneficial in polymyositis and dermatomyositis resistant to other therapy.

PROGNOSIS

- Inflammation is usually active for 2–3 years.
- Treatment with corticosteroids and other immunosuppressants produces improvement of symptoms in around 75% of patients.
- Complete recovery occurs in 20%.
- Mortality after several years of active disease is roughly 15%.

11.6 MUSCULAR DYSTROPHIES

DEFINITIONS

- Group of inherited muscle disorders characterized by muscle weakness and wasting.

DYSTROPHINOPATHIES

- Dystrophin is a component of the muscle cell membrane connecting the cell to the extracellular matrix and is essential for normal muscle function.
- Major types:
  - Duchenne muscular dystrophy (DMD);
  - Becker muscular dystrophy (BMD);
- see **Table 11.1**.

MICRO-facts

Gower's sign

- Gower's sign is a commonly described symptom of proximal weakness in children with dystrophinopathies.
- To stand up from the floor, the child 'walks' his or her hands up the legs and bodies. This compensates for weakness in the proximal muscles instead of relying on the stronger distal muscles of the arms.

Table 11.1 **Comparison of Duchenne's and Becker's muscular dystrophy**

	DMD	BMD
Aetiology	• Gene for dystrophin is found on the X chromosome; mutations of dystrophin therefore most commonly affect males who have only one copy of the gene.	
Pathophysiology	• Production of dystrophin protein is prevented.	• Partially functional form of dystrophin protein produced.
Clinical features	• Usually presents by age 5 • Cardiomyopathy • Cognitive impairment	• Usually presents between ages 8 and 25 but can appear later • Cardiomyopathy – rarely • Cognitive impairment – rarely
	• Proximal muscle weakness (e.g. Gower's sign; see MICRO-facts) • Calf pseudohypertrophy (replacement of muscle with fatty tissue, causing calves to appear enlarged) • Joint contractures: develop within a few years of onset of symptoms	

(Continued)

Table 11.1 (Continued)

	DMD	BMD
Investigations	• CPK raised	• CPK may be raised (to lesser extent than DMD)
	• DNA analysis identifies mutation in dystrophin gene in around 70% of cases. • Negative DNA test does not rule out the diagnosis as a mutation may be undetectable in up to 30% of affected individuals. • Muscle biopsy and dystrophin analysis may be required, particularly when genetic testing is negative.	
Management	• **Genetic counselling**: Female family members may be investigated for carrier status with a serum CPK measurement (mildly raised in carriers) or DNA analysis if the mutation is known. • **Regular physiotherapy** helps to prevent the formation of joint contractures. • **Surgical treatment** may be considered for secondary scoliosis. • **Drug treatment** (e.g. corticosteroids) may be used to indirectly defer disease progression by increasing muscle strength. • **Ventilatory support** (e.g. bi-level positive airway pressure, BiPAP) may be useful as respiratory failure develops.	
Prognosis	• Median survival 35 years. • Usually unable to walk by age 10 years.	• Variable severity. • Many maintain ability to walk and have nearly normal life expectancy.

Neurological zones

> **MICRO-print**
>
> **Other muscular dystrophies**
> - **Facioscapulohumoral dystrophy:**
>   - Autosomal dominant inheritance is present.
>   - Progressive weakness affecting ocular muscles and muscles of the face, neck and shoulder girdle occurs. Winging of the scapula is prominent. Eventually, leg muscles are involved and patients may develop foot drop.
>   - Serum CPK usually is normal or mildly raised.
>   - Severity of symptoms is highly variable; some patients are confined to a wheelchair early on; others notice only mild weakness in old age.
> - **Limb-girdle dystrophy:**
>   - This presents as a diverse group of autosomal dominant, autosomal recessive and X-linked muscle disorders with a wide variation in clinical presentation.
>   - The most common symptom is a slowly progressive proximal muscle weakness similar to the dystrophinopathies, but note that in many forms, both genders will be affected equally.

> **MICRO-print**
>
> Treatment of the inherited muscular dystrophies is primarily supportive. However, advances in research of the underlying genetic defects makes them good candidates for developments in gene therapies. In mouse models of DMD, there has been significant success with introduction of a plasmid containing the unmutated dystrophin gene.

11.7 MYOTONIC DYSTROPHY

DEFINITION

- Myotonic dystrophy is an inherited, highly variable multisystem disorder characterised by muscle wasting and myotonia.
- Myotonia is the delayed relaxation of muscle fibres following stimulation.

AETIOLOGY

- Autosomal dominant condition:
  - **Type 1**: more common form; caused by a pathologically expanded trinucleotide repeat sequence in the *DMPK* (myotonic dystrophy protein kinase) gene. Like other triple-repeat disorders, anticipation is a feature.

- **Type 2**: caused by a pathologically expanded tetranucleotide repeat sequence in the *ZNF9* (zinc finger protein 9) gene; does not show anticipation.

EPIDEMIOLOGY

- **Prevalence**: approximately 5 per 100,000.
- Most common muscular dystrophy in adults.

PATHOPHYSIOLOGY

- Clinical myotonia occurs due to electrical hyperexcitability of individual muscle fibres.
- The mechanisms of pathogenesis of the two mutations causing myotonic dystrophy are proposed to involve RNA processing.

CLINICAL FEATURES

- **Weakness and wasting**:
  - **Type 1**: involving facial muscles (including ptosis), bulbar muscles and distal limb muscles.
  - **Type 2**: involving proximal muscles.
- **Myotonia**: an inability to relax after performing a movement. Myotonia is demonstrated clinically as:
  - **Grip myotonia**: inability to relax the hand muscles after gripping an object, such as when shaking hands.
  - **Percussion myotonia**: percussion of the belly of a muscle, such as the thenar eminence, produces a dimple that slowly 'refills' as the muscle relaxes.
- Premature cataract formation;
- Cognitive impairment;
- Cardiovascular conduction abnormalities such as first-degree heart block and bundle branch block are more common in type 1 myotonic dystrophy.

> ## MICRO-facts
> The characteristic myotonic facies of type 1 myotonic dystrophy is produced by ptosis and facial muscle weakness combined with frontal balding.

INVESTIGATIONS

- **Electromyography**: There is repeated firing of muscle fibre action potential following a stimulus and a decrease in amplitude and frequency of action potentials over time.
- **Genetic testing**: Identification of a pathological repeat sequence allows confirmation of the diagnosis.

Neurological zones

MANAGEMENT

- **Genetic counselling**: Family members of affected individuals should be offered genetic testing.
- **Drug treatment**:
  - Phenytoin can be used to improve myotonia if this is a major problem.
  - There is no available drug treatment for the muscular weakness.
- **Ventilatory support**: As respiratory failure develops, ventilatory support may be useful.
- **Cardiovascular monitoring**: Affected individuals should have annual electrocardiograms (ECGs).
- Physiotherapy, occupational therapy and speech therapy should be provided.
- Cataract surgery may be necessary.

11.8 ENDOCRINE AND TOXIC MYOPATHIES

ENDOCRINE MYOPATHIES

- Endocrine abnormalities may produce a proximal weakness; treatment in each case is to correct the underlying endocrine abnormality.
- **Thyrotoxicosis**: In the majority of patients, weakness develops after onset of thyrotoxic symptoms.
- **Hypothyroidism**: Weakness is usually mild. It is associated with painful cramping and slow-relaxing reflexes.
- **Glucocorticoid excess** (steroid myopathy):
  - Excess glucocorticoids, due to either Cushing's syndrome or exogenous steroid use, can produce an endocrine myopathy.
  - Fluorinated steroids (betamethasone and dexamethasone) are more likely to cause myopathy.
  - Steroid myopathy without other features of steroid excess (e.g. weight gain, easy bruising, etc.) is unlikely.

TOXIC MYOPATHIES

Alcoholic myopathy

- **Acute necrotising myopathy**: Acute necrotizing myopathy can develop over several days following an 'alcoholic binge'. It is characterized by weakness, myalgia, muscle swelling, and a marked rise in the serum CPK. Spontaneous recovery will occur with avoidance of alcohol.
- **Chronic myopathy**: Long-term heavy alcohol consumption can produce a slowly progressive proximal myopathy with wasting. Alcohol abstinence can improve symptoms over several months.

Drug-induced myopathies

- Many drugs can cause muscle damage, ranging in severity from mild serum CPK elevation with no symptoms to acute rhabdomyolysis.
- Stopping the suspected drug usually results in resolution of symptoms.
- Commonly used drugs known to cause myopathy include **statins, fibrates, cyclosporin** and **zidovudine**.

Part III

Neurological disorders

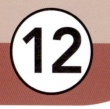

Cerebrovascular disease

12.1 STROKE

- Stroke is defined as a vascular insult producing rapid onset of neurological deficit:
    - **stroke**: neurological disturbance lasting longer than 24 hours;
    - **transient ischaemic attack (TIA)**: neurological disturbance that resolves completely within 24 hours.
- It is the third most common cause of death in the United Kingdom after heart disease and cancer and second leading cause of disability worldwide.
- Stroke results from either **ischaemia** or **haemorrhage**; ischaemia is the more common pathological process.
- Other related disorders may produce symptoms that do not fit with the accepted definition of stroke but have a vascular basis: subdural haematoma (SDH)/extradural haematoma (EDH), venous sinus thrombosis.

12.2 ISCHAEMIC STROKE AND TRANSIENT ISCHAEMIC ATTACK

Definition

- The rapid onset of focal neurological deficit as a result of an occluded arterial supply.

Epidemiology

- Accounts for 80% of all strokes.
- **Incidence**: There are 240 per 100,000 population per year in the United Kingdom.
- **Age**: Incidence increases with advancing age.

Aetiology

- **Thrombosis**: Rupture of an atherosclerotic plaque leads to thrombosis and sudden vessel occlusion.
- **Microembolism**:
    - Usually, there is a cardiac source (e.g. thrombus) (atrial fibrillation [AF] most common cause) or valvular vegetations in endocarditis.

- Venous microemboli may occlude cerebral vessels if a conduit between right and left heart exists (e.g. patent foramen ovale).
- **Other vascular causes**: fibromuscular dysplasia, arterial dissection, vasculitis, venous sinus thrombosis.
- **Cardiac**: low cardiac output/systemic blood pressure (BP) (e.g. cardiac arrhythmias); cardiac source of emboli (see previous discussion of microembolism).
- **Haematological**: thrombocytosis, polycythaemia, sickle cell disease, hypercoagulability.

Pathophysiology

- Arterial supply to an area of neurological tissue is occluded; if collateral blood supply is inadequate, tissue ischaemia occurs, resulting in focal neurological deficit.
- If cerebral perfusion is not rapidly reestablished, infarction will result.
- Neurological recovery in a TIA occurs when blood flow is restored by autoregulation within the brain; vasodilation of vessels means infarction is avoided, and the neurological deficit is thus transient.

MICRO-facts

Risk factors for ischaemic stroke

- Smoking.
- Diabetes mellitus.
- Hypertension.
- Hypercholesterolaemia.
- Family history of atherosclerotic disease in relatives under 65 years.

Clinical features

- Depend on the arterial territory affected.
- **Anterior circulation**:
  - contralateral hemiparesis;
  - hemisensory loss;

MICRO-print
Neglect

- Neglect involves damage to the area of the brain containing an internal map of the area of space around the subject's own body.
- Neglect produces apparently strange phenomena, such as the denial of ownership of certain limbs or an inability to comprehend events or objects to one side of the body.

continued…

continued...

- Note that neglect is related to attention and not vision; patients can observe any object but simply fail to comprehend the part of the object on the side of the neglect.
- Neglect is particularly common in the early phase after a stroke; fortunately, it rarely lasts beyond this initial period.

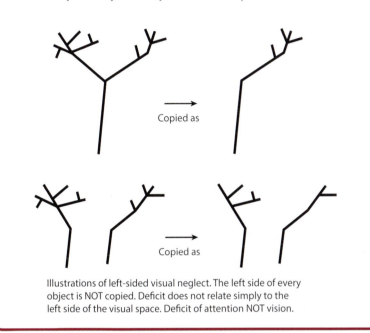

Illustrations of left-sided visual neglect. The left side of every object is NOT copied. Deficit does not relate simply to the left side of the visual space. Deficit of attention NOT vision.

   - expressive or receptive dysphasia (if the dominant hemisphere is affected);
   - homonymous hemianopia.
- **Posterior circulation**:
   - unilateral/bilateral/alternating paresis or sensory loss;
   - ipsilateral cerebellar symptoms (e.g. ataxia) (see Chapter 6 for more details);
   - features of **brainstem stroke**:
      – cranial nerve palsies, often ipsilateral;
      – quadriplegia;
      – locked-in syndrome;
      – brainstem infarction syndromes (see Section 3.7, MICRO-print).
- Typically, symptoms of TIA last only minutes to hours; however, they can last up to 24 hours.

MICRO-facts

Features of TIA

Rather than the focal neurological deficits described, a TIA may present with **amaurosis fugax**:

- transient monocular blindness due to involvement of the ophthalmic branch of the anterior cerebral artery, causing monocular field loss.

MICRO-print

Bamford classification of stroke

The Bamford classification of stroke gives an indication of stroke territory and likely prognosis:

- **Total anterior circulation stroke (TACS)** includes all three of the following:
  - contralateral hemiparesis or contralateral hemisensory loss;
  - contralateral homonymous hemianopia;
  - cortical defects (e.g. expressive or receptive dysphasia).
- **Partial anterior circulation stroke (PACS)** requires two of the three features of a TACS.
- **Posterior circulation stroke (PoCS)** includes one or more of the following features:
  - cranial nerve palsies;
  - cerebellar symptoms;
  - isolated homonymous hemianopia (i.e. without other features of a TACS or PACS).
- **Lacunar stroke** involves occlusion of penetrating branches of the middle and anterior cerebral arteries, which supply deep grey matter and white matter. A **lacunar** stroke will present with **one** of the following:
  - isolated contralateral hemiparesis;
  - isolated contralateral hemisensory loss;
  - contralateral hemiparesis and ataxia, with the ataxia out of proportion to the weakness.
- **'Dysarthria – clumsy hand syndrome'**: dysarthria associated with ataxia and weakness of the contralateral hand.

A TACS carries the worst prognosis, with only 5% of patients independent at 1 year; for PoCS, PACS and lacunar strokes, the equivalent figure is approximately 60%.

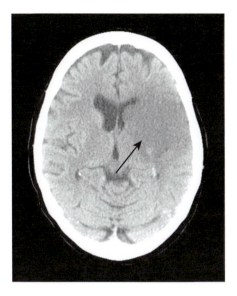

Fig. 12.1 CT image showing left middle cerebral artery (MCA) territory stroke.

INVESTIGATIONS

- Full examination is important not only to detect symptoms of stroke but also to identify a possible cause.
- **Brain imaging**:
  - **computed tomography (CT)**: vital to detect haemorrhagic stroke; may not detect small or early ischaemic lesion (see **Fig. 12.1**);
  - **magnetic resonance imaging (MRI)** with diffusion-weighted imaging (DWI): best available investigation for identifying ischaemic strokes, particularly those that may not be visible on CT (early/small lesions, posterior fossa stroke).
- **Basic blood investigations**:
  - full blood count, lipid profile, blood glucose, and inflammatory markers;
  - **younger patients**: full thrombophilia screen and an autoantibody screen for vasculitis.
- **Cardiac investigations**: electrocardiogram (ECG), echocardiogram.
- **Carotid Doppler**: to identify carotid stenosis.

MANAGEMENT OF TIA

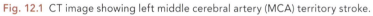

- **Risk assessment**: assess the risk of a subsequent ischaemic stroke using **ABCD2 score** (see MICRO-print following).
- Patients with greater than 70% carotid stenosis on the side supplying the affected hemisphere should be considered for carotid endarterectomy or carotid stenting.

Neurological disorders

- **Antiplatelet medication**:
  - Give 300 mg of aspirin (given immediately once CT head has ruled out haemorrhage).
  - Current U.K. guidelines suggest clopidogrel after stroke and aspirin and dipyridamole after TIA. It is likely that as newer anti-platelets come on to the market, guidelines will change.
- **Hypertension management**: Aim for a BP less than 140/85 mmHg.
- **Hypercholesterolaemia**: Statins reduce the risk of stroke even if cholesterol is within normal limits.

MICRO-print

ABCD2 score to calculate seven-day stroke risk in TIA

- **A**ge: greater than 60 years: +1 point.
- **B**lood pressure: greater than 140 mmHg systolic or greater than 90 mmHg diastolic: +1 point.
- **C**linical features:
  - unilateral weakness: +2 points;
  - speech disturbance without weakness: +1 point;
  - other signs: 0 points.
- **D**uration of symptoms:
  - longer than 60 minutes: +2 points;
  - 10–59 minutes: +1 point.
- **D**iabetes present: +1 point.

Add the points to obtain a total (maximum of 7):

- **Score 0–4:** The 7-day risk is 0.4%. Urgent outpatient follow-up (1–2 weeks) is needed.
- **Score 5:** The 7-day risk is 12%. Urgent investigation within 24 hours is needed.
- **Score 6:** The 7-day risk is 31%. Admit for monitoring and urgent investigation.

MANAGEMENT OF ISCHAEMIC STROKE

- Admit to a specialist stroke unit.
- **Thrombolysis** with recombinant tissue plasminogen activator (e.g. alteplase) should be considered within 4.5 hours of symptoms:
  - Haemorrhagic stroke must be excluded on CT head.
  - Check for other contraindications, including recent surgery, head injury and other anti-coagulants.
  - There is significant risk of cerebral haemorrhage.

- Antiplatelet medication, carotid assessment and BP modification as for TIA.
- Anticoagulation considered if source of embolism identified (e.g. AF; see the following MICRO-facts).
- Swallowing assessment should be performed before giving any oral hydration, food or medication; consider alternative hydration/feeding routes in the interim.

MICRO-print

The CHADS$_2$ score, based on the presence of several risk factors, is used to calculate the risk of thromboembolic stroke in patients with AF:

C	Congestive heart failure	1 point
H	Hypertension (BP > 140/90)	1 point
A	Age > 75	1 point
D	Diabetes	1 point
S$_2$	Previous stroke/TIA	2 points

The CHA$_2$DS$_2$Vasc score is a refinement of this, using additional risk factors:

C	Congestive heart failure	1 point
H	Hypertension (BP > 140/90)	1 point
A$_2$	Age >75	1 point
D	Diabetes	1 point
S$_2$	Previous stroke/TIA	2 points
V	Vascular disease	1 point
A	Age 64–75	1 point
Sc	Sex (female gender)	1 point

The total number of points indicates the risk of thromboembolic stroke and whether formal anticoagulation is indicated:

0 points	low risk: no treatment or aspirin
1 point	moderate risk: aspirin or oral anticoagulant (usually warfarin)
2+ points	high risk: oral anticoagulant

Neurological disorders

- **Rehabilitation**
  - Of stroke survivors, 40% are left with a degree of functional impairment.
  - A multidisciplinary process involving physiotherapy, occupational therapy and speech therapy is used.
  - Consideration of mood, cognitive function, continence, functional ability, pain and communication is needed.
  - Comprehensive package of community care should be provided.

MICRO-print

Carotid artery dissection

- A tear the wall of the carotid artery, which leads to an intramural haematoma and subsequent microemboli, producing **anterior circulation ischaemic stroke**.
  - May occur spontaneously or following **trauma**. Rapid deceleration in a road traffic incident is a common cause.
  - Cause of stroke in all age groups, including **young people**.
- Onset may be associated with **neck pain**; expansion of the carotid artery can affect the sympathetic chain and lead to **Horner's syndrome**.
- Carotid artery dissection is usually identified by **magnetic resonance arteriography**.
- Similarly, **vertebral artery dissection** may produce a posterior circulation ischaemic circulation stroke.

MICRO-case

Ischaemic stroke

Mrs R is a 74-year-old woman who lives in a residential home. She is on treatment for hypertension and has long-standing paroxysmal AF. One morning, she complains that she is unable to get out of bed due to weakness of her left leg; the residential home staff also find her difficult to understand. They call for an ambulance, and she is taken to the emergency department.

When she is seen in the emergency department, she is noted to be slightly confused but denies any headache, neck stiffness or photophobia. She cannot see the doctor properly when he is standing on her left side. Her daughter arrives and says that Mrs R was fine when she saw her yesterday.

On examination, Mrs R is noted to have reduced tone and power in her left arm and leg, with the weakness more pronounced in the arm. The reflexes are absent on the left but normal on the right. She has dysarthria, but no dysphasia, and left-sided facial weakness. She also has

continued...

continued...

a left upper homonymous quadrantanopia, but examination of the fundi is unremarkable. She has reduced sensation over her left arm and leg.

An urgent CT scan of the brain is requested, and this shows no abnormality. MRI with DWI is then performed; this shows an area of infarction in the right middle cerebral artery territory. As the time of onset of Mrs R's symptoms cannot be established, she is not thought to be a good candidate for thrombolytic therapy. She is admitted to the stroke unit and commenced on secondary prevention.

After several days, on repeat examination Mrs R is noted to have increased tone in her left arm and leg, with clasp knife rigidity in the left arm. Power remains reduced in both the left limbs. Her reflexes on the left side are brisk, and her plantars are extensor on the left side and flexor on the right. The rigidity and weakness of her limbs slowly improves with physiotherapy, and her other symptoms also become better over the course of her admission. She is eventually discharged to her residential home with some residual weakness in her left arm, but otherwise makes a full recovery.

Summary points

- Ischaemic stroke may initially produce a flaccid paralysis that becomes spastic over several days. Upper motor neuron signs also develop, including brisk reflexes and extensor plantars.
- Prompt brain imaging is required in all cases of suspected stroke.
- CT is better at detecting haemorrhage early, although MRI, particularly with DWI, is better at identifying areas of infarction.
- In ischaemic stroke, thrombolysis must be commenced within 4.5 hours of the onset of symptoms. Immediate brain imaging is needed to rule out intracerebral haemorrhage.

12.3 INTRACRANIAL HAEMORRHAGE

DEFINITION

- Any bleed within the cranial cavity, including subarachnoid haemorrhage (SAH) and subdural, extradural and parenchymal haemorrhage.

MICRO-print

Intracranial pressure in intracranial haemorrhage

Intracranial bleeds are important because bleeding into the rigid cranial cavity has potential to cause a lethal increase in **intracranial pressure (ICP)**.

A key component of management of intracranial bleeds is thus monitoring the ICP, with urgent intervention if levels become too high.

Neurological disorders

MICRO-print

Head injury

Head Injury is common and an important cause of **intracranial haemorrhage**. However, head injury can cause morbidity and mortality by mechanisms other than haemorrhage, such as diffuse axonal injury. Haemorrhage is important to consider as intervention in a timely manner may prevent further damage to the brain.

Assessment of the patient with a head injury involves identifying patients at a higher risk of intracranial haemorrhage who should have CT imaging of the brain and skull. Indications for **CT scanning** are as follows:

- more than **one** episode of vomiting;
- **Glasgow Coma Scale (GCS) score less than 13** when first assessed in the hospital;
- GCS less than 15 **2** hours after injury;
- suspected **skull fracture**; look for signs of a base-of-skull fracture (i.e. haemotympanum, 'panda' eyes, CSF leakage from ears or nose, Battle's sign);
- **seizure** following head injury;
- focal neurological deficit;
- **amnesia** of events more than 30 minutes before head injury.

In addition, patients who have experienced any amnesia or loss of consciousness following a head injury, even if they do not meet the criteria mentioned, should have a CT scan if they are over **65** years old, have a history of **coagulopathy** or there was a particularly **dangerous** mechanism of injury.

SUBARACHNOID HAEMORRHAGE

DEFINITION

- Bleeding into the cerebrospinal fluid (CSF)-containing subarachnoid space.

AETIOLOGY

- Trauma.
- Spontaneous rupture of a berry aneurysm (80% of spontaneous SAHs).
- Arterial-venous malformations.

- Coagulopathy.
- Rupture of a mycotic aneurysm (may complicate infective endocarditis).
- Occasionally idiopathic.

PATHOPHYSIOLOGY

- **Berry (or saccular) aneurysms**:
  - intracranial arteries prone to 'outpouching' and aneurysm formation;
  - arterial walls relatively unsupported by external structures, so increases the likelihood of rupture;
  - most common site for formation is the circle of Willis.

MICRO-print

Berry aneurysms

Berry aneurysms may occur in isolation, or they may be associated with a familial clinical syndrome. The most common examples are **autosomal dominant polycystic kidney disease (ADPCKD)** and **Ehlers–Danlos syndrome**. A patient with ADPCKD **and** a family history of aneurysms should be screened for aneurysms using magnetic resonance angiography.

CLINICAL FEATURES

- Sudden-onset severe headache ('thunderclap headache'), which is usually occipital.
  - Usually reported as 'worst headache imaginable'.
- Features of raised ICP.
- **Meningism**: photophobia, neck stiffness and positive Kernig's sign.
- Transient loss of consciousness or reduced level of consciousness.
- Seizures (approximately 6% of patients).

INVESTIGATIONS

- **Blood tests**:
  - Screen for coagulopathy and to detect complications such as hyponatraemia (see complications below);
  - Hypomagnesaemia is a marker of poor prognosis.
- **CT brain**: detects approximately 95% of SAH.
- **Lumbar puncture**: should be performed if the CT head is normal.

> **MICRO-print**
> **Lumbar puncture in SAH**
>
> - Xanthochromia describes the yellow appearance of CSF due to red blood cell degradation and release of bilirubin.
> - Lumbar puncture must be performed **12 hours** after the onset of symptoms to allow the breakdown of red blood cells.
> - Detection of xanthochromia differentiates a SAH from the introduction of small amounts of blood as a result of trauma during the procedure ('traumatic tap').
> - The CSF sample must be protected from light to avoid degradation of red cell breakdown products.

- **CT angiography**: performed after SAH is confirmed to localise aneurysms and arteriovenous malformations prior to intervention.

MANAGEMENT

- Transfer to a neurosurgical unit:
  - Patients have a high risk of complications or further bleeding.
  - Active management is focused on trying to prevent further bleeding or complications occurring.
- **Medical management**:
  - **Nimodipine**: used to reduce vascular tone and prevent cerebral ischaemia as a result of vasospasm;
  - **BP control**: aim for systolic BP of 130–140 mmHg (intravenous agents may be used);
  - Avoid stimuli that may increase ICP; strict bed rest with sedation if required. If features of raised ICP are present:
    - intubate and ventilate;
    - maintain pCO_2 in the range 4–4.5 kPa to reduce risk of hyperventilation-associated vasospasm;
    - may administer mannitol to reduce ICP.
  - Analgesia for headache and antiemetics as required.
- **Surgical management**: appropriate if an anatomical cause of SAH is identified that is amenable to modification to prevent further episodes:
  - **Aneurysm occlusion**: clipping the neck of the aneurysm or inserting a metallic coil to fill the aneurysm and thus prevent blood flow into it;
  - **Arterial-venous malformations**: can be treated with direct surgery, radiosurgery or endovascular embolisation.

COMPLICATIONS

- Rebleeding is common in the days following a SAH.

- Cerebral ischaemia may occur secondary to raised ICP or days afterwards as a result of cerebral vasospasm.
- Seizures.
- Cardiopulmonary dysfunction (e.g. cardiogenic pulmonary oedema).
- SIADH (syndrome of inappropriate anti-diuretic hormone secretion): causes hyponatraemia associated with high urinary sodium and high urinary osmolality. It is a common complication of both SAH and neurosurgical intervention.

PROGNOSIS

- Prognosis is dependent on age, location of aneurysm and the clinical condition on admission to hospital.
- Of these patients, 30–40% die in the first few days.
- SAH secondary to an arteriovenous malformation has a better prognosis than an aneurysmal bleed.

SUBDURAL HAEMATOMA

- Most often caused by blunt head trauma.
- Forms when the bridging veins that drain the venous sinuses are ruptured.
- In the elderly and some other groups such as alcoholics, cerebral atrophy makes the bridging veins more susceptible to damage.
- An SDH may present **acutely** or **chronically** with altered cognition over a period of weeks; thus, SDH is part of the differential diagnosis for new-onset confusion.
- An SDH will form a crescent-shaped collection of blood over one hemisphere on CT of the head.
  - The haematoma does not cross the midline as bound by falx cerebri (see Section 3.6).
- See **Fig. 12.2**.

EXTRADURAL HAEMATOMA

- Usually occurs when fracture of the temporal or parietal bone causes a tear of the middle meningeal artery.

CLINICAL FEATURES

- Head trauma followed by loss of consciousness.
- Later followed by a period of lucidity and then deterioration as the haematoma expands.
- An EDH is contained by strong dural attachments to the skull and forms a localised biconvex shape on CT head; midline shift may be evident with compression of ventricles.

Neurological disorders

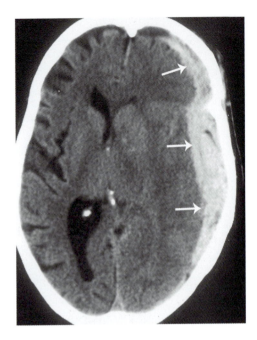

Fig. 12.2 CT image showing subdural haematoma.

- Surgical drainage of an EDH is required urgently.
- See **Fig. 12.3**.

PARENCHYMAL HAEMORRHAGE

- Bleeding into the brain parenchyma occurs for a number of reasons, some of which are amenable to secondary prevention:
  - hypertension;
  - trauma;
  - amyloid angiopathy;
  - microbleeds;
  - intracranial neoplasm;
  - coagulation disorders most commonly related to anticoagulant therapy.
- The distribution of the bleed gives clues:
  - Deep-seated bleeds such as within the basal ganglia are typical of hypertensive bleeds.
  - Larger bleeds within the cortex, which may be multiple in elderly patients, are suggestive of amyloid angiopathy.
- Angiography should be performed if there is any doubt regarding the aetiology:
  - after 6 weeks (allows the haematoma to resolve);
  - to detect underlying arteriovenous malformation or cavernoma that could rebleed.

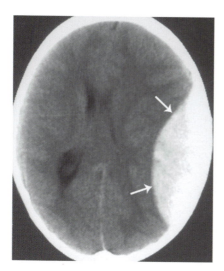

Fig. 12.3 CT image showing frontal extradural haematoma.

- May be amenable to treatment with either surgery or radiotherapy:
  - Mass effect of haemorrhage and associated cerebral oedema leads to a rise in ICP; methods to reduce ICP are often required, including decompressive craniotomy.
- See **Table 12.1**.

MICRO-print

Stroke and anticoagulation therapy

Patients on **anticoagulant therapy** with an intracranial bleed are a special case:

- Warfarin (or other vitamin K antagonist anticoagulants) should be stopped immediately and intravenous **vitamin K** administered. This should be accompanied by **Beriplex** 30 IU/kg by slow intravenous injection (Beriplex is a combination of clotting factors II, VII, IX, X and proteins C and S).

Following an ischaemic stroke, any anticoagulant therapy should be withheld for at least 6 weeks as there is a significant risk of haemorrhagic transformation in the infarcted area of tissue.

12.4 VENOUS SINUS THROMBOSIS

DEFINITION

- Thrombus formation within the intracranial venous system, producing neurological deficit.

Neurological disorders

Neurological disorders

Table 12.1 Features of intracranial haemorrhages

HAEMATOMA TYPE	AETIOLOGY	VESSEL INVOLVED	CT APPEARANCE
Subarachnoid haemorrhage	• Trauma • Rupture of a berry aneurysm • Arteriovenous malformation • Coagulopathy • Rupture of mycotic aneurysm	• Circle of Willis	• Increased attenuation may be seen over the cerebral hemispheres, ventricles or CSF spaces.
SDH	• Blunt head trauma	• Bridging veins	• Crescent-shaped, high-density lesion with a concave surface lying away from the skull.
EDH	• Fracture of temporal or parietal bone	• Middle meningeal artery (most common)	• Bi-convex, high-density lesion. • Spread limited by dural adhesion to skull.
Parenchymal haemorrhage	• Trauma • Hypertension • Intracranial neoplasm • Amyloid angiopathy	• Small penetrating intracerebral vessels	• High-density area on CT scan. • Traumatic bleeds tend to occur in temporal, frontal or occipital poles, where sudden deceleration of the head causes the brain to impact on bony prominences.

PATHOPHYSIOLOGY

- Thrombosis within the venous sinuses results in tissue ischaemia due to venous congestion and indirectly via a rise in ICP.
- This most commonly occurs in the superior sagittal sinus, followed by the lateral sinus and the cavernous sinus.

AETIOLOGY

- Usually occurs in the context of a hypercoagulable state.
- Antiphospholipid syndrome: may occur in isolation or in conjunction with **connective tissue** disease.
- Primary or secondary polycythaemia.
- Nephrotic syndrome.
- Oestrogen-based hormone therapy (oral contraceptive pill or hormone replacement therapy).
- Pregnancy and the puerperium.
- Infection: may complicate otitis media, sinusitis, meningitis, or a cerebral abscess.
- Trauma.

CLINICAL FEATURES

- Severe headache:
  - Headaches can precede the onset of focal neurological deficit by several weeks.
  - Occasionally, a sudden-onset headache is described, but more often, the headache is 'throbbing' or 'tight' in character.
- Symptoms of raised ICP, including papilloedema and vomiting, are present.
- Seizures may occur.
- The pattern of focal neurological deficit is variable depending on the site of the thrombosis:
  - Hemiparesis may occur on the contralateral side to the thrombosis.
  - Cranial nerve palsies are common.
  - **Superior sagittal sinus thrombosis**: associated with paraparesis due to compression of both motor cortices.
  - **Cavernous sinus thrombosis**:
    - This is associated with ipsilateral periorbital oedema, exophthalmos and papilloedema.
    - Cranial nerves III, IV, VI and V (ophthalmic branch) run through the cavernous sinus, and thrombus formation can result in palsy.
    - This pattern of neurological deficit should prompt investigation for cavernous sinus thrombosis.

INVESTIGATIONS

- **Blood investigations**: Full blood count, complete thrombophilia screen, autoantibody screen.

- **Brain imaging**:
  - CT or MRI with or without venography should be performed.
  - Identification of an area of infarction that does not correspond to an arterial supply should raise the suspicion of venous sinus thrombosis.

MANAGEMENT

- Treat any underlying cause.
- Anticonvulsants for seizures.
- Anticoagulation:
  - Treat with heparin initially and then warfarin.
  - If secondary haemorrhage is present on imaging, then caution should be exercised.
- **Surgical intervention**:
  - Surgery is indicated for severe neurological deterioration.
  - A thrombus can be removed and local thrombolysis administered.

PROGNOSIS

- At 16 months, approximately 88% of patients make a total or near-total recovery.
- Mortality is approximately 10%.

MICRO-facts

Glasgow Coma Scale

- **Best motor response:**
  6. Obeying commands/spontaneous.
  5. Localising response to pain.
  4. Withdraws to pain.
  3. Flexor response to pain.
  2. Extensor posturing to pain.
  1. No response to pain.

- **Best verbal response:**
  5. Oriented.
  4. Confused conversation.
  3. Inappropriate speech.
  2. Incomprehensible speech.
  1. None.

- **Eye opening:**
  4. Spontaneous eye opening.
  3. Eye opening in response to speech.
  2. Eye opening in response to pain.
  1. No eye opening.

Score 13–15 indicates mild injury; 9–12, moderate injury; 8 or less, severe injury.

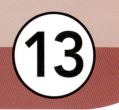

13 Intracranial tumours

13.1 OVERVIEW

DEFINITION
- Benign or malignant growth within the cranial cavity.
- Most commonly a secondary metastasis from a distant primary malignancy.

CLINICAL FEATURES
- Presentation varies depending on the tumour type and its location.
- Features include:
  - raised intracranial pressure (ICP);
  - new-onset focal seizures (with or without secondary generalisation) in an adult;
  - neurological deficit (variable depending which area of the brain is affected).

INVESTIGATIONS
- **Diagnostic imaging**:
  - Magnetic resonance imaging (MRI) is superior for identifying lesions, particularly in the posterior fossa.
  - Definitive imaging with computed tomography (CT) or MRI requires pre- and post-contrast scans, although some tumours may be visible on a plain scan (e.g. a calcified meningioma).
- A biopsy or resection specimen is required to confirm the diagnosis in cases of primary brain tumours.

MANAGEMENT
- Surgical resection.
- Radiotherapy may be used alone if surgical resection is not possible or as an adjunct to surgery.
- Chemotherapy is used to palliate and to lengthen survival.
  - It can be delivered orally, intravenously or even directly into the central nervous system (CNS) via wafers placed into a post-surgical cavity.
- **Medical**:
  - Anticonvulsants are used to manage seizures.
  - Corticosteroids help reduce associated oedema.

13.2 MENINGIOMA

DEFINITION

- A primary tumour arising from any part of the meninges.

PATHOPHYSIOLOGY

- May be familial; some associated with neurofibromatosis type II.
- Extensive vascular supply and a tendency to calcify.
- Most benign and slow growing.

INVESTIGATIONS

- **CT or MRI brain with contrast**: If a meningioma is extensively calcified, it may be visible on a plain scan (see **Fig. 13.1**).

MANAGEMENT

- **Asymptomatic**: observe as these are likely to be slow growing.
- **Symptomatic**: surgical resection followed by biopsy for histology.
- Corticosteroids may be used pre- and post-operatively.

PROGNOSIS

- Prognosis depends on the grade of the tumour and the degree of surgical resection achieved.
- Around 10% of completely resected low-grade tumours reoccur within 10 years.

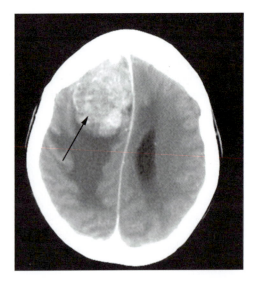

Fig. 13.1 CT scan (with contrast) showing a frontal meningioma.

13.3 GLIOMA

DEFINITION

- A glioma is a benign or malignant tumour arising from glial (support) cells in the brain or, less commonly, in the spinal cord.
- The most common is a high-grade astrocytoma, also known as **glioblastoma multiforme**. These are aggressive tumours, and life expectancy is usually months if untreated (also occur as transformed low-grade tumours).
- New seizures in the context of a low-grade 'benign' tumour can herald transformation into a higher, more aggressive grade.

PATHOPHYSIOLOGY

- May be associated with the neurocutaneous syndromes (see Chapter 18).
- The type of glioma depends on the glial cell population giving rise to the tumour:
    - **astrocytoma**: arises from astrocytes; most common type of glioma;
    - **ependymoma**: arises from the epithelial lining of the ventricular system of the brain and spinal cord;
    - **oligodendrogliomas**: from oligodendrocytes (glial cells responsible for insulating nerve axons – analogous to Schwann cells in the peripheral nervous system [PNS]).
- **Mixed gliomas**: contain more than one subtype of glial cell.

MANAGEMENT

- Surgical removal or debulking:
    - Functional MRI may allow more tumour to be removed by mapping out eloquent areas (such as motor and speech centres).
    - Awake craniotomy to test function or intraoperative MRI can improve tumour debulking.
- Newer chemotherapeutic regimes have also increased survival.

13.4 HEMANGIOBLASTOMA

DEFINITION

- Benign tumour arising from vascular tissue within the CNS.

AETIOLOGY

- Sporadic.
- Familial: Von Hipple–Lindau syndrome:
    - autosomal dominant inheritance;
    - associated with haemangioblastomas in the CNS, kidney and eye.

Neurological disorders

CLINICAL FEATURES

- Variable depending on the tumour location.
- May be a long history of minor symptoms followed by a sudden exacerbation.

MANAGEMENT

- Symptomatic haemangioblastomas should be treated by surgical resection.

13.5 PITUITARY NEOPLASIA

AETIOLOGY

- Comprises 10–15% of intracranial tumours, most commonly non-functioning adenomas, but may produce any of the anterior pituitary hormones (prolactin, growth hormone, adrenocorticotrophic hormone [ACTH], thyroid-stimulating hormone [TSH], luteinizing hormone/follicle-stimulating hormone [LH/FSH]).
- Most commonly affect young adults.

CLINICAL FEATURES

- **Mass effects**:
  - Bitemporal hemianopia is via compression of the optic chiasm (see **Fig. 8.1**).
  - CSF rhinorrhoea is due to extension into the sphenoid sinuses.
  - Lateral extension can lead to compression of the cavernous sinuses and their contained structures; this can cause diplopia due to cranial nerve palsy and ophthalmoplegia.
- **Hormonal effects**:
  - Excess hormone production by the tumour:
    - Excess prolactin is the most common syndrome and produces amenorrhea, infertility and galactorrhoea in women; may present subtly in men with decreased libido and impotence.
    - Acromegaly is due to growth hormone excess.
    - Cushing's disease is due to excess ACTH secretion.
  - Hormone deficiency (due to obliteration of one or more compartments of the pituitary gland):
    - Gonadotrophin deficiency may result in oligo-/aemonorrhea, impotence, infertility;
    - TSH deficiency: hypothyroidism (may be masked by a coincident deficiency of ACTH, which produces a non-specific lack of energy and weight loss).

INVESTIGATIONS

- MRI.
- Formal visual field testing.

MANAGEMENT

- Medical treatment of endocrine abnormalities:
  - A prolactinoma is initially treated medically with a dopamine agonist (e.g. cabergoline), which corrects the prolactin levels and shrinks the tumour.
  - Hormone replacement may be required.
- Surgical resection can be performed, usually via a trans-sphenoidal approach.
- Radiotherapy may be required if surgical resection is incomplete.

PROGNOSIS

- Remission is achieved in 90% of patients with a microadenoma (a tumour < 1 cm in diameter) and 50–60% of patients with a macroadenoma (tumour > 1 cm in diameter).

MICRO-facts

Pituitary apoplexy

- Acute haemorrhage into the pituitary occurs, usually due to a pituitary tumour. In 80% of cases, the tumour has not been diagnosed previously.
- This presents as a sudden-onset headache associated with rapid onset of pituitary mass effect due to the expanding haematoma (e.g. visual loss and diplopia).
- Patients subsequently develop deficiency of the various pituitary hormones (panhypopituitarism).

MICRO-case

Cerebral neoplasia

A 63-year-old postman presents to the acute neurology ward with a history of headaches. On questioning, the patient has been experiencing daily headaches for the past 3 months that are now interfering with his work.

They are worse in the morning, and he often vomits on waking. The headaches gradually improve over the day but seem to return when straining or bending down. Over the past week, he has had three periods of visual blurring, which lasted for approximately 2 minutes, following some heavy lifting. He has not noticed any weakness of his arms or legs or new-onset confusion but has felt very tired lately.

His past medical history includes type II diabetes mellitus (diet controlled), and he has recently given up smoking but smoked for 60 pack-years. He occasionally drinks alcohol.

continued...

Neurological disorders

continued...

Systemic enquiry reveals a persistent dry cough for the past year and unexplained weight loss of 1 stone over the past 6 months.

On examination, he has some dullness to percussion of his right lung base but normal cardiovascular and gastrointestinal examination. His neurological examination reveals limited abduction of his left eye and diplopia on left lateral gaze. Venous pulsations are absent on fundoscopy. There are no other focal neurological signs.

You order a set of bloods, a chest X-ray and a CT head to determine the cause of his symptoms.

Unfortunately, the results show a well-defined opacity in the right lung with an associated pleural effusion. There is also a mass in the left hemisphere of the brain.

A further CT thorax/abdomen/pelvis is ordered to stage the cancer.

The patient is diagnosed with a secondary brain metastasis from a lung primary cancer.

Summary points

- A detailed history and examination are imperative in patients with neurological signs; it can be very easy to miss related underlying pathology.
- Patients with serious underlying pathology can present with subtle symptoms.
- The most common cause of intracranial tumour is secondary metastasis from a primary malignancy elsewhere.

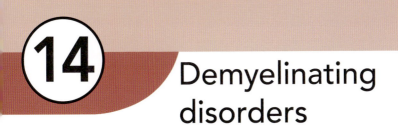

14 Demyelinating disorders

14.1 MULTIPLE SCLEROSIS

DEFINITION

- Multiple sclerosis (MS) is an autoimmune disease that targets myelinated neurons in the central nervous system (CNS), resulting in focal disturbance of function that is often transient.
- Disease pattern differs between affected individuals and stages of the disease.

EPIDEMIOLOGY

- **Prevalence**: 100–120 per 100,000 people in Western Hemisphere. MS is less prevalent in equatorial regions.
- **Age**: Average age of onset is 30 years.
- **Gender**: Females affected more than males (approximately 2:1).
- **Genetic factors**:
  - Modest effect in MS; concordance rate in monozygotic twins about 20–35%.
  - Association with human leucocyte antigen (HLA)-DR15 and DQ6; HLA-DRB1 may be protective.

PATHOPHYSIOLOGY

- CNS damage is via a T-cell-mediated immune response, which produces localised plaques of demyelination in the white matter throughout the CNS.
  - Damage to both the axon and myelin sheath of targeted nerves also occurs.

CLINICAL FEATURES

- Formation of a demyelinating plaque in the CNS leads to a corresponding focal neurological deficit, which is often monosymptomatic (e.g. weakness, numbness or tingling in one or more limbs or unilateral optic neuritis).
- MS is classified by the pattern of symptom progression:
  - **Relapsing-remitting (RRMS)** (80% of patients at onset): Successful remyelination occurs between episodes of demyelination. Patients typically experience monosymptomatic neurological deficit with complete recovery between episodes.

- **Secondary progressive**: Most patients with RRMS will eventually develop cumulative loss of function with increasing disability between acute relapses. (About 65% of patients with RRMS develop secondary progressive MS after 15 years.)
- **Primary progressive (PPMS)** (10–15% of patients): Chronic progressive demyelination from disease onset produces cumulative loss of function. This is more common in patients who develop MS late (>45 years old).

MICRO-facts

PPMS is characterised by episodes of neurological deficit that are **separated in space and time**. There are very few other pathologies that produce recurrent transient neurological disease in spatially separated areas of the CNS.

- Focal neurological deficit in MS can take almost any form depending on the location of a demyelinating plaque in the CNS. Common presentations include the following:
    - **Optic neuritis**: Subacute visual loss or blurring occurs, usually with central scotoma and pain on eye movement.
    - **Transverse myelitis**: Features are as for any spinal cord injury, with neurological deficit below the level of the lesion commonly including a sensory level and spastic paraparesis. Magnetic resonance imaging (MRI) typically shows a high T2-weighted lesion less than one spinal segment in length.
    - **Internuclear ophthalmaplegia (INO)**: INO is caused by a plaque affecting the medial longitudinal fasciculus (MLF).
        - The MLF connects the ipsilateral III nucleus with the contralateral VI nucleus to allow coordinated horizontal eye movement.
        - A patient with INO will exhibit a failure of eye adduction on the affected side along with nystagmus of the contralateral abducting eye.
        - Diplopia is a common presenting complaint.
        - Convergence is preserved (i.e. the eye is able to adduct successfully when the MLF is not required).
        - INO in a younger person is almost pathognomonic for MS; in older patients, stroke is a more common cause.
    - **Sensory symptoms**: Positive or negative sensory symptoms may occur.
    - **Lhermitte's sign** is particularly characteristic: A lesion in the cervical dorsal column produces electric shock sensations in the spine, legs and occasionally arms on sudden neck flexion.
    - **Cerebellar signs** include ataxic gait and clumsy hands.
    - **Facial weakness**: MS may produce a lower motor neuron pattern of facial weakness.

MICRO-facts

Uhthoff's phenomenon

In Uhthoff's phenomenon, about 25% patients with MS report that their symptoms are transiently worsened by exercise or heat (such as a hot bath). Typically, symptoms appear with the trigger and then settle after 20–30 minutes.

MICRO-print

Neuromyelitis optica/Devic's disease

- Neuromyelitis optica (NMO) or Devic's disease is an autoimmune condition closely related to MS. It is caused by autoantibodies directed against aquaporin 4, a water-conducting protein expressed by astrocytes.
- **Clinical features:** Demyelinating plaques affect the optic nerve and the spinal cord:
  - The lesions are similar but not identical to those in MS, but often more severe: Transverse myelitis extends more than three spinal segments (one in MS); optic neuritis is often bilateral.
  - NMO often presents with optic neuritis and transverse myelitis occurring in rapid succession. Such a presentation should prompt testing for anti-aquaporin 4 antibodies alongside MS investigations.
  - Some patients suffer only a single episode, but most experience successive relapses.
- **Management:**
  - Acute episodes are treated with intravenous methylprednisolone; plasma exchange may be required.
  - Immunosuppression with azathioprine or alternative agents is used for prevention of attacks.
  - Beta interferon is not effective in NMO.
  - Recovery between relapses in NMO does not tend to be complete as in RRMS; patients experience increasing disability with successive relapses.

INVESTIGATIONS

- **Imaging**:
  - MRI is sensitive for detecting areas of demyelination and useful for excluding differential diagnoses.
  - T2-weighted images show white matter lesions (lesions that enhance with contrast represent active disease).

Neurological disorders

- The combination of enhancing and non-enhancing lesions suggests that lesions are separated in time and space.
- **Cerebrospinal fluid (CSF) analysis**:
  - Oligoclonal bands of immunoglobulin (IgG) on electrophoresis may be found in approximately 95% of MS patients at some stage. They must be absent from serum to imply primary CNS inflammation.
  - Note that oligoclonal bands may also be present in other inflammatory disorders of the CNS.
  - Slight lymphocytosis and minimally elevated protein may also be present.
- **Neurophysiology**: Used to detect asymptomatic CNS demyelination, neurophysiology is rarely used now that MRI is easily accessible. The principle of each test is to demonstrate delayed conduction of a nerve impulse suggestive of demyelination:
  - **Visual evoked potentials (VEP)**: A visual stimulus is provided, and electrical activity is recorded over the visual cortex to look for evidence of optic neuritis.
  - **Somatosensory evoked potentials**: A sensory stimulus is provided, and electrical activity is recorded through sensory pathways to look for demyelination in white matter tracts.

MICRO-print
Revised MacDonald diagnostic criteria for MS

CLINICAL PRESENTATION	ADDITIONAL DATA NEEDED
2 or more attacks (relapses) **OR** 2 or more objective clinical lesions	None; clinical evidence suffices (additional evidence desirable but must be consistent with MS)
2 or more attacks **OR** 1 objective clinical lesion	Dissemination in space, demonstrated by MRI **OR** positive CSF and two or more MRI lesions consistent with MS **OR** a further clinical attack involving a different site
1 attack **OR** 2 or more objective clinical lesions	Dissemination in time, demonstrated by two or more MRI scans **OR** a second clinical attack

continued...

continued...

1 attack **OR** 1 objective clinical lesion (monosymptomatic presentation)	Dissemination in space demonstrated by MRI **OR** positive CSF and two or more MRI lesions consistent with MS **AND** dissemination in time demonstrated by two or more MRI scans **OR** a second clinical attack
Insidious neurological progression suggestive of MS (PPMS)	One year of disease progression (retrospectively or prospectively determined) **AND** two of the following: (1) positive brain MRI (nine T2 lesions or four or more T2 lesions with positive VEP); (2) positive spinal cord MRI (two focal T2 lesions); (3) positive CSF

MANAGEMENT

- **Acute relapses**:
  - To minimise steroid exposure, treatment is indicated only if functional deficit occurs.
  - Oral prednisolone or high-dose intravenous methylprednisolone is an appropriate choice.
  - Steroids shorten relapses but do not affect prognosis.
  - Steroid-non-responsive relapses may be treated with plasma exchange.
- **Disease-modifying therapy**:
  - **Beta-interferon** and **glatiramer acetate**:
    - Both reduce the rate of relapse by 30% in active RRMS.
    - Both treatments are administered by subcutaneous/intramuscular injection.
    - Patients must have had at least two significant relapses within the past 2 years to qualify for treatment.
    - Neither treatment is shown to improve the long-term prognosis of MS.
  - **Natalizumab**:
    - This is a monoclonal antibody against the Very Late Antigen-4 (VLA-4) receptor (normally allows immune cells to adhere to and cross the blood-brain barrier).
    - Natalizumab is administered monthly by intravenous infusion.
    - Shown to reduce relapses in RRMS by two-thirds and MRI lesions by around 90%.
    - Reactivation of JC virus infection to produce progressive multifocal leucoencephalopathy is a significant adverse effect.

Neurological disorders

- **Mitoxantrone**:
  - Mitoxantrone is a cytotoxic immunosuppressant agent licensed for secondary progressive MS.
  - Side effects include a risk of cardiotoxicity and lymphoma.
- **Symptomatic treatment**:
  - Spasticity may be ameliorated with baclofen (orally or via an intrathecal pump in very severe cases).
  - Detrusor instability may be treated with anticholinergic medication or catheterisation.
  - Various agents are available for the treatment of neuropathic pain.
- Involvement of a multidisciplinary team (physiotherapists, occupational therapists, speech and language therapists and psychologists) is an important component of MS management.

MICRO-facts

Intercurrent infection will worsen neurological symptoms in MS. It is therefore important to perform a **septic screen** to differentiate infection from acute relapse as a cause of acute deterioration; the administration of immunosuppression in infection is unlikely to be helpful and may be harmful.

PROGNOSIS

- Poor prognostic factors include the following:
  - male gender;
  - increased age at time of onset;
  - primary progressive disease;
  - widespread disease at onset (assessed either clinically or by MRI);
  - less than 1 year between the first two relapses of a relapsing-remitting course.
- Median time to death is approximately 30 years from onset.

14.2 ACUTE DISSEMINATED ENCEPHALOMYELITIS

DEFINITION

- Acute disseminated encephalomyelitis (ADEM) is an autoimmune demyelinating disorder of the CNS; it follows a monophasic course (unlike MS) and is most often post-infective (or after recent vaccination or very rarely organ transplantation).

EPIDEMIOLOGY

- Incidence is approximately 8 per million and is most common in children and adolescents (can occur at any age).

PATHOPHYSIOLOGY

- ADEM is thought to be due to T-cell-mediated autoimmune response (as in MS).
- Differences between ADEM and MS are possibly due to the particular cytokines and chemokines mobilized.
- ADEM appears to be a post-infective event: An immune response is mobilized against a component of an invading pathogen, which is then active against a similar component of the host.

CLINICAL FEATURES

- Onset usually is within 1–20 days of an infective illness or vaccination.
- At onset of neurological symptoms, patients have usually completely recovered from their preceding illness.
- The onset of neurological features is usually over a few days. Symptoms are diffuse and may include any of the descriptions of neurological deficit in MS.
- Encephalopathy is often present, and patients may suffer seizures.

INVESTIGATIONS

- MRI shows multiple asymmetric white matter plaques representing active demyelination.
- CSF examination shows elevation of white cell counts; however, CSF electrophoresis is usually negative for oligoclonal bands (more suggestive of MS).

MANAGEMENT

- Treatment is most often with intravenous methylprednisolone or intravenous immunoglobulin (IVIG).
- Possible alternatives include cyclophosphamide and plasma exchange.

PROGNOSIS

- Most patients make a full recovery with minimal or no neurological deficit. The 10-year risk of developing MS is approximately 25%.

14.3 OTHER DEMYELINATING DISEASES

PROGRESSIVE MULTIFOCAL LEUCOENCEPHALOPATHY

- See Section 19.5.

Neurological disorders

CENTRAL PONTINE MYELINOLYSIS

- Central pontine myelinolysis is a symmetric non-inflammatory demyelination in the pons.
  - It occurs as a complication of rapid correction of hyponatraemia.
  - Severe hyponatraemia should be corrected at a rate of no more than 8–10 mmol/l of sodium per day.
- Clinical features are of brainstem demyelination with cranial nerve dysfunction (commonly pseudobulbar palsy or gaze palsies) and spastic quadriplegia.
- There is no specific treatment; therefore, the emphasis is on prevention. Prognosis is poor, and some patients may develop a locked-in syndrome as a result of their severe neurological deficit.

LEUCODYSTROPHIES

- Leucodystrophies are a group of disorders in which there is white matter loss due to dysmyelination (whereby the normal development of myelin is disrupted by inborn errors of metabolism) or demyelination.
- These disorders usually present in infancy/childhood with severe neurological deficit and early death, but there are adult-onset leucodystrophies.
- These conditions are often undiagnosed, and some are only diagnosed at post-mortem.
  - Identification of enzyme deficiency or abnormal metabolic products in blood or urine may allow diagnosis.
- Management is frequently supportive only; prognosis varies according to the specific disorder, but most are fatal in childhood.

VITAMIN B$_{12}$ DEFICIENCY

- See Section 9.7.

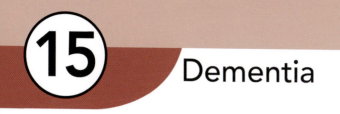

15 Dementia

15.1 GENERAL OVERVIEW

DEFINITION

- Dementia is an impairment of cognitive function sufficient to cause a loss of social functioning in a previously unimpaired person.
- Onset and progression of dementia occurs over months to years.
- Dementia is distinct from delirium (see the MICRO-facts on page 180).

> **MICRO-facts**
>
> The onset of dementia is over an extended period of time, usually without sudden change. A collateral history is often necessary to establish the course of cognitive decline.

INVESTIGATIONS

- The degree and pattern of cognitive impairment should be identified by a careful history, cognitive screening (e.g. Mini-Mental State Examination, MMSE) and formal neuropsychological testing:
    - The MMSE is commonly used but is poor at detecting early dementia or mild cognitive impairment (MCI) as it does not test anterograde memory very well.
    - Newer tests such as the Addenbrooke's cognitive examination are better at detecting MCI.
- Patients with suspected dementia should be investigated to rule out any reversible causes of dementia or delirium (see **Table 15.1**).
    - **Imaging**: Magnetic resonance imaging (MRI) of the brain is more sensitive than computed tomography (CT) of the head at detecting lobar atrophy. It may detect other intracranial abnormalities (e.g. bleeding or tumour).
    - **Blood investigations**:
        - See **Table 15.2**.
        - Genetic testing for familial Alzheimer's disease (AD) or Huntington's disease may be appropriate.

Table 15.1 Causes of dementia

	CAUSE OF DEMENTIA	PROMINENT CHARACTERISTICS
Degenerative	• Alzheimer's disease	• Memory loss, language impairment, depression/anxiety, delusions
	• Frontotemporal dementia	• Frontal: personality/behavioural change • Temporal: language impairment
	• Lewy body dementia and Parkinson's disease and dementia	• Parkinsonism, visual hallucination prominent
	• Progressive supranuclear palsy and corticobasal degeneration	• Parkinsonism, motor disturbance
	• Creutzfeld-Jakob disease	• Rapidly progressive dementia with myoclonus
	• Huntington's disease	• Chorea, psychiatric disturbance
Vascular	• Vascular dementia	• Dementia, typically subcortical with executive dysfunction plus focal neurological deficit, stepwise decline
	• Vasculitis	• Systemic illness, features of connective tissue disease
	• Chronic subdural haematoma	• History of trauma
	• CADASIL (see text)	• Dementia preceded by stroke at young age
Infective	• HIV encephalopathy	• Was previously associated with AIDS but is now recognized in HIV; may respond to antiretroviral with good CSF penetrance
	• Progressive multifocal leucoencephalopathy (PML)	• Caused by JC virus and associated with HIV infection; features white matter lesions on MRI; no treatment other than HAART if HIV positive
	• Neurosyphilis	• Argyll-Robertson pupil, tabes dorsalis, prominent psychotic symptoms

Malignancy	• Primary intracranial tumours • Cerebral metastases • Paraneoplastic and autoimmune encephalitidies	• Notable focal neurological deficit; raised intracranial pressure; primary neoplasm may be evident elsewhere, especially breast/lung • Presence of autoantibodies (e.g. anti-Hu, anti-VGKC and anti-glutamate receptor)
Hydrocephalus	• Normal-pressure hydrocephalus	• Urinary incontinence, gait disturbance
Metabolic	• Chronic renal failure • Hypothyroidism • Addison's disease • Hepatic encephalopathy • Vitamin B$_{12}$ deficiency • Wilson's disease • Porphyria	• Other features of primary organ failure • Macrocytic anaemia, polyneuropathy, leg weakness (SACD) • Kayser-Fleischer rings, cirrhosis, extrapyramidal signs, family history • Peripheral neuropathy, abdominal pain, family history
Trauma	• Trauma	• History of preceding head injury
Psychiatric	• Pseudodementia	• Cognitive impairment occurring in the context of depression

HAART, highly active antiretroviral therapy; VGKC, voltage-gated potassium channel; SACD, subacute combined degeneration (of the spinal cord)

- **Cerebrospinal fluid (CSF)** examination may be helpful if infection or CJD (Creutzfeld–Jakob disease; protein 14-3-3) is suspected.
- **Electroencephalogram (EEG)** if CJD or seizures is a possibility.

Table 15.2 Rationale for investigations in dementia/delirium

TEST	CORRESPONDING REVERSIBLE CAUSE OF DEMENTIA/DELIRIUM
Full blood count	Macrocytosis in vitamin B_{12} deficiency, raised white cell count in infection
Erythrocyte sedimentation rate (ESR) and C-reactive protein (CRP)	Raised in infection and vasculitis
Urea and electrolytes	Abnormal renal function possible in acute or chronic renal failure; abnormal electrolytes an important cause of delirium
Glucose	Low in hypoglycaemia
Thyroid function	Abnormal in hypo-/hyperthyroidism
Haematinics	Vitamin B_{12} deficiency an important cause of dementia
Autoimmune screen	Vasculitis/connective tissue disease
Serology	HIV/syphilis

MICRO-facts

Delirium is an **acute-onset confusional state**. Unlike dementia, delirium is usually **reversible**.

	DELIRIUM	DEMENTIA
Onset	Sudden	Gradual
Course	Usually fluctuating	Usually progressive (may be fluctuating in some forms)
Level of consciousness	Often impaired (may be agitated or drowsy/withdrawn)	Normal (until late disease)
Prominent cognitive deficits	Attention, concentration	Memory, language difficulties
Progression/duration	Improves with treatment of underlying cause; may persist for days/weeks/months	Cognitive decline may be slowed with medication; however, this is a chronically progressive condition.

GENERAL PRINCIPLES OF MANAGEMENT

- **Pharmacological**:
  - Routine use of sedation should be avoided; however, it is sometimes necessary to allow essential investigations to be performed.
  - Cognitive enhancers (acetylcholinesterase inhibitors, NMDA [N-methyl-D-aspartate] receptor antagonists) can produce symptomatic benefit and may slow the decline in cognition in certain forms of dementia (see Section 5.2).
- **Non-pharmacological**:
  - Patients with dementia are often unable to adequately self-care and will need assessment of their activities of daily living.
  - Patients with severe dementia often need 24-hour care in a residential or nursing home.

15.2 ALZHEIMER'S DISEASE

DEFINITION

- Degenerative disorder causing progressive cognitive decline with prominent memory impairment.
- It is the most common cause of dementia, accounting for 50% of all cases.

PATHOPHYSIOLOGY

- AD produces generalised cortical atrophy, which is most prominent in the temporal lobes.
- It is characterised histopathologically by extracellular amyloid plaques and intracellular neurofibrillary tangles consisting of aggregated tau protein.

AETIOLOGY

- Most cases are idiopathic.
- Approximately 0.1% of cases are familial, with autosomal dominant inheritance.
  - Familial cases usually present at a younger age than sporadic cases. Causal mutations have been identified in the amyloid precursor protein gene, presenilin 1 and presenilin 2.
  - Risk of developing disease (including sporadic) and age at onset are related to number of apolipoprotein E ε-4 alleles.

EPIDEMIOLOGY

- **Gender**: females more affected than males.
- **Incidence**: increases with age. Annual incidence estimated at 0.6% for persons aged 65–69 but 8.4% for persons aged greater than 85.

Neurological disorders

CLINICAL FEATURES

- Progressive cognitive impairment occurs over 7–10 years.
    - **Memory loss** is prominent. Typically, it affects episodic memory (e.g. what they had for breakfast) and anterograde memory (formation of new memories); long-term memory is also affected later.
    - **Language difficulties** are characterised by a reducing vocabulary.
    - **Apraxia** is the inability to execute complex movements despite having the desire and the necessary physical ability (can lead to a risk of falling). This is due to the involvement of the parietal lobe.
    - **Agnosia** is the loss of ability to recognise objects or people.

INVESTIGATIONS

- See investigations discussion in Section 15.1. CT head shows generalised atrophy, particularly in the temporal and parietal lobes.
- SPECT (single-photon emission computed tomography) is shown to be superior to other imaging in differentiating AD from other forms of dementia.
- Diagnosis is based on the pattern of cognitive impairment and the absence of another diagnosis. Definitive diagnosis is at post-mortem by histopathology.
- Genetic testing is done if familial disease is suspected (see the discussion of aetiology in this section).

MANAGEMENT

- **Non-pharmacological**: A multidisciplinary team (MDT) approach, including assessment by physiotherapists, occupational therapists and a social worker, is crucial.
- **Pharmacological**: No drug has been shown to provide a significant reduction in cognitive decline:
    - Acetylcholinesterase inhibitors (donepezil, galantamine and rivastigmine) are licensed for the treatment of AD.
    - The NDMA receptor antagonist memantine is indicated in moderate disease if a patient is unable to tolerate one of the other drugs and is recommended in severe disease.
    - Antipsychotics are avoided if possible but may be required for treatment of prominent behavioural or psychiatric features.

PROGNOSIS

- The mean life expectancy from diagnosis is 7 years; in their last year, patients often require 24-hour nursing care.

15.3 DEMENTIA WITH LEWY BODIES

DEFINITION

- Dementia with Lewy bodies (DLB) is a degenerative disorder producing a progressive dementia associated with parkinsonism.
- It is distinguished from Parkinson's disease-associated dementia (PDD) by the onset of cognitive symptoms in tandem, or within a year, of the motor symptoms.

PATHOPHYSIOLOGY

- Similar to both Parkinson's disease and AD:
  - **Lewy bodies** are alpha-synuclein cytoplasmic inclusions found in neurons of the cerebral cortex and brainstem. They are also found in Parkinson's disease, and both diseases feature a loss of dopaminergic neurons from the substantia nigra.
  - Generalised brain atrophy with amyloid plaques and neurofibrillary tangles occurs in up to 50% of cases; this suggests it may be a variant of AD.

EPIDEMIOLOGY

- Second most common dementia, accounting for 10–15% of cases.
- **Gender**: males greater than females.
- **Incidence**: estimated at 0.1% annually.
- **Age**: most patients between 50 and 85 years old at disease onset.
- The majority of DLB cases are sporadic rather than familial.

CLINICAL FEATURES

- Progressive cognitive impairment with marked fluctuation. Memory is usually preserved in early stages, but there is prominent impairment of attention and alertness.
- Psychotic features can occur, including delusions and visual hallucinations.
- **Parkinsonism**: resting tremor, bradykinesia, rigidity and a shuffling gait (falls being more prominent than in early AD).

INVESTIGATIONS

- See Section 15.1; CT/MRI head show generalised atrophy (temporal lobe atrophy less marked than in AD).

MANAGEMENT

- Use of dopaminergic medication to ameliorate the Parkinsonian symptoms of DLB can worsen the psychotic features; equally, the use of antipsychotic medication can worsen the Parkinsonian symptoms.

Neurological disorders

- Patients with DLB also have a high incidence of neuroleptic malignant syndrome in response to antipsychotic medication.
- Acetylcholinesterase inihibitors may be of benefit.
- An MDT approach is used.

PROGNOSIS

- No disease-modifying treatment is currently available.
- Average survival from diagnosis is 8 years.

15.4 FRONTOTEMPORAL DEMENTIA (PICK'S DISEASE)

DEFINITION

- Frontotemporal dementia (Pick's disease) is a degenerative disorder causing progressive cognitive decline with prominent personality and language disturbance.

PATHOPHYSIOLOGY

- Marked cerebral atrophy occurs, predominantly affecting the frontal and temporal lobes.
- It is histopathologically characterised by tau-, TDP-43- or fus-containing intracellular deposits.

AETIOLOGY

- There is likely a strong genetic element; approximately 50% of patients with frontotemporal dementia have a family history of dementia.
- Pathogenic mutations are identified in a number of genes including those coding for Tau and progranulin.
- Some mutations suggest a degree of overlap with motor neuron disease

EPIDEMIOLOGY

- **Gender**: females greater than males.
- **Age**: onset usually between 40 and 60 years old.
- **Prevalence**: estimated to be low, approximately 5 per million population.

CLINICAL FEATURES

- Onset is usually early compared to other forms of dementia.
- Different clinical syndromes occur depending on primary site of brain degeneration:
  - **Frontal lobes**: Progressive personality change is prominent: loss of motivation, concentration and changes in moral attitude, emotional lability and aggressive behaviour.

- **Temporal lobes**: Patients gradually lose the meaning in their speech, such that their speech may be fluent but nonsensical (semantic dementia) or gradual loss of speech fluency (primary progressive aphasia).
- Memory impairment is not prominent

INVESTIGATIONS

- See Section 15.1 (MMSE does not perform well in identifying frontal lobe dysfunction.)
- **CT/MRI head**: shows severe frontotemporal atrophy.

MANAGEMENT

- No treatment has been demonstrated to be effective in frontotemporal dementia; emphasis is on supportive care.

PROGNOSIS

- Death usually occurs between 5 and 10 years after diagnosis.

15.5 VASCULAR DEMENTIA

DEFINITION

- Process by which recurrent vascular events can cause cumulative damage to the cerebral cortex, resulting in progressive cognitive decline.
    - Stroke and vascular disease can accelerate the presentation of dementia in patients with underlying AD pathology.

EPIDEMIOLOGY/PATHOPHYSIOLOGY

- Related to cerebrovascular disease:
    - any intracranial haemorrhage (parenchymal/extra-parenchymal);
    - cerebrovascular infarction or small-vessel ischaemia;
    - vasculitis;
    - hereditary forms such as CADASIL (cerebral autosomal dominant angiopathy and stroke ischaemic leucodystrophy).

CLINICAL FEATURES

- Pattern of cognitive deficit depends on the site of ischaemic damage (e.g. language is impaired in temporal lobe damage).
- Often associated with other neurological signs of cerebrovascular damage (although may be absent).
- Classically 'step-wise' progression of cognitive decline due to successive vascular events (contrast with steady decline in other forms of dementia).

Neurological disorders

INVESTIGATIONS

- Full assessment should be made for vascular risk factors.
- **CT/MRI head**: Mild atrophy may be present. Areas of infarction can be visualised, particularly on MRI.
- Genetic testing for mutations in the notch gene is available for the diagnosis of CADASIL.

MANAGEMENT

- Aggressive management of vascular risk factors.

PROGNOSIS

- Prognosis is variable but dependent on effective modification of atherosclerosis risk factors.
- Survival is approximately 8 years from diagnosis.

MICRO-case

Alzheimer's disease

A 67-year-old retired accountant presents to the general practitioner (GP) as her husband is becoming increasingly concerned about her recent unusual behaviour.

She has become increasingly forgetful over the past year, often going to the supermarket and forgetting numerous items; she even forgot her husband's birthday this year. She went to the local shops yesterday and rang her husband as she was unable to find her way home, despite having visited these shops many times before.

She has always been fiercely independent with lots of hobbies; however, a few close friends have commented that she has appeared withdrawn recently.

She is otherwise well and has no past medical history. On examination, her respiratory, cardiovascular and gastrointestinal examinations are normal. She has no focal neurological signs but performed poorly on the MMSE, scoring only 17/30. In particular, she struggled with drawing and on subtracting serial sevens.

She is admitted to the hospital for further testing. All her blood tests, urine dipstick and chest X-ray are normal, and her lumbar puncture shows less than 1 white cell and less than 1 red blood cell. Her MRI shows excessive atrophy that is not in keeping with her age.

A diagnosis of AD is made. She is started on donepezil, and an MDT review is performed to identify and address needs of the patient and her husband.

continued…

continued...

Summary points

- Patients with AD present with progressive cognitive decline, often with prominent memory disturbance.
- It is important to consider the implications on family members when a diagnosis of dementia is made. Early referral to occupational therapy and social services is important to maintain independence.

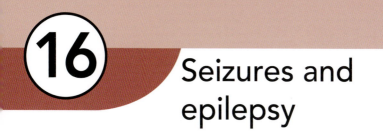

Seizures and epilepsy

16.1 OVERVIEW

DEFINITION

- **Seizures**:
    - excessive or hypersynchronous brain activity producing transient disturbance in brain function or reduced consciousness;
    - may manifest as sensory or, more often, motor symptoms.
- **Epilepsy**: recurrent unprovoked seizures.

EPIDEMIOLOGY

- **Prevalence**:
    - lifetime prevalence of a single seizure about 10% (significant proportion are febrile convulsions);
    - lifetime prevalence of epilepsy 1.5–5%.

PATHOPHYSIOLOGY

- Can be caused by anything that results in neuronal hyperexcitability, including chemical or metabolic imbalance and structural or ischaemic damage to brain tissue.
- Various stimuli lower the seizure threshold in individuals with an existing predisposition:
    - sleep deprivation;
    - infection;
    - alcohol;
    - metabolic disturbance (e.g. hypoglycaemia, hypernatraemia, hypomagnesaemia and hypocalcaemia).

AETIOLOGY

- Sixty per cent of seizures are idiopathic.
- **Neurological disorders**:
    - febrile convulsions in children (increased risk of subsequent seizures if prolonged or recurrent);
    - cerebral dysgenesis (cerebral palsy, arteriovenous malformation [AVM], Sturge–Weber syndrome);

- space-occupying lesion, including neoplasia;
- head trauma;
- stroke;
- infections.
- **Systemic/metabolic disorders**:
  - hypoglycaemia;
  - hyponatraemia;
  - hypocalcaemia;
  - uraemia;
  - hepatic encephalopathy;
  - porphyria;
  - drug/alcohol withdrawal;
  - eclampsia;
  - hyperthermia.

INVESTIGATIONS

- **Blood tests**: FBC, U&Es, Ca^{2+}, liver function tests (LFTs) and blood glucose.
- **Septic screen**, including inflammatory markers, chest X-ray and urinalysis.
- **Brain imaging**: initially computed tomography (CT), magnetic resonance imaging (MRI) is better at identifying structural abnormalities.
- **Electroencephalography (EEG)**:
  - Abnormalities are seldom detectable between seizures, so in isolation an EEG is a poor test to diagnose epilepsy.
  - EEG is useful for diagnosing subtypes of epilepsy once a clinical diagnosis has been made.
  - Video telemetry with EEG during an attack is diagnostic and is the gold standard method for identifying seizure subtypes (may be normal in simple partial seizures).
  - It is only practical if patients are having very frequent seizures (i.e. several per week) as most admissions are for 3 or occasionally 5 days.

MANAGEMENT

- Most seizures are self-terminating and short lasting. Generalised tonic-clonic seizures usually last less than 90 seconds and do not require abortive treatment.
- Aim of management is preventing or at least reducing the frequency of seizures (medication, lifestyle modification).
- Prolonged or recurrent seizures should be managed as status epilepticus.
- Precipitating cause should be corrected if possible.
- Management of epilepsy (i.e. unprovoked seizures) is dependent on the seizure type and patient.

COMPLICATIONS

- Status epilepticus.
- Sudden unexpected death in epilepsy (SUDEP): annual incidence approximately 0.5% in refractory epilepsy.

PROGNOSIS

- By 12 months, 60–70% of patients will be seizure free with anticonvulsant therapy.

16.2 CLASSIFICATION OF SEIZURES

GENERALISED SEIZURES

- Generalized seizures result from abnormal electrical activity affecting the entire cerebral cortex. The structure of the brain looks normal, and there is no focal start to seizures.
- **Tonic-clonic**: Both can occur individually as well as together. There are several distinct phases:
  - **Tonic phase: (lasts < 1 minute)**:
    - There is stiff extension of the limbs and neck and loss of consciousness.
    - Breathing ceases, and patient may become cyanosed.
  - **Clonic phase (lasts several minutes)**:
    - There is rhythmic alternating contraction and relaxation of limb muscles.
    - Irregular breathing occurs; patient may remain hypoxic.
    - Tongue biting and urinary incontinence may occur.
  - **Coma** (lasts several minutes – related to length of tonic-clonic period):
    - Clonic movements subside, but the patient remains unconscious.
    - Hypoxia resolves as breathing becomes normal.
  - **Confusion/post-ictal** (lasts minutes to hours):
    - The patient may remain confused and drowsy for a significant period after the seizure.
- **Absence seizures**:
  - Patients become temporarily unresponsive, often adopting a 'staring-into-space' posture.
  - Facial automatisms may occur, such as repetitive blinking.
  - Limbs remain still (no convulsion or loss of postural tone).
  - A seizure lasts less than 10 seconds; the attack ends suddenly, and there is no post-ictal phase.
  - Patients are often unable to identify that they have had an attack.
  - Patients may experience several attacks per day.

Neurological disorders

- **Myoclonic jerks**:
  - These are abrupt arrhythmic muscle jerks that most commonly affect upper limbs.
  - They are not usually associated with a loss of consciousness and last less than a second.
  - Myoclonic jerks may cluster or even evolve into a clonic seizure.
  - Myoclonic jerks during the onset of sleep are a normal phenomenon.
- **Atonic seizures**:
  - There is brief loss of muscle tone, which often results in falls with significant injury.

FOCAL SEIZURES (PARTIAL SEIZURES)

- **Focal seizures**:
  - These seizures involve abnormal activity in a specific region of the brain.
  - Abnormal activity may spread to involve the entire cerebral cortex, producing a generalised seizure (**secondary generalisation**).
- **Simple focal seizures**: Consciousness is retained.
  - Symptoms depend on the area of the cortex involved; these are classified as motor, sensory, autonomic or psychic.
  - A 'Jacksonian march' refers to a progression of clonic movements from distal to proximal muscles, reflecting progression of abnormal electrical activity across the primary motor cortex.
  - Simple focal seizures of the temporal lobe are characterised by abnormal sensation, for example, taste, smell or amnestic disturbances such as déjà vu.
- **Complex focal seizures**: Impaired consciousness.
  - Involve either the frontal lobe or the temporal lobe;
  - Often preceded by an aura;
  - Usually with motor automatisms:
    - **temporal lobe**: lip smacking, chewing or hand fumbling;
    - **frontal lobe**: bizarre motor symptoms such as bicycling or a fencing posture.
  - Post-ictal confusion is often brief relative to a generalised seizure.
- **Todd's paresis**: focal neurological deficit that persists after resolution of a focal or tonic-clonic (i.e. generalised) seizure for up to 36 hours.

STATUS EPILEPTICUS

- Textbook definition of *status epilepticus* is a continuous seizure lasting more than 30 minutes or repeated seizures without recovery of consciousness.
- In practice, a seizure lasting longer than 10 minutes would normally be treated as status epilepticus. This is important as response to treatment diminishes with time.

- Causes are as for any seizure; often, it is associated with poor compliance or acute withdrawal of anti-convulsant therapy.
- Status epilepticus often consists of a generalised tonic-clonic seizure, but any type of seizure may evolve into status epilepticus.
  - A prolonged absence seizure may be difficult to differentiate from another cause of unresponsiveness.
- Investigations are as for any seizure; if the diagnosis is in doubt, EEG is useful.
- **Emergency management**:
  - **Ensure airway is patent** (may require airway adjuncts or intubation). Place patient in recovery position. High-flow 100% oxygen should be administered with or without suction.
  - **Abortive treatment**:
    - A slow intravenous bolus is given of 4 mg **lorazepam**, followed by a second dose after 10 minutes if there is no response.
    - Outside the hospital, buccal midazolam or rectal diazepam is used.
    - If seizures persist, a **phenytoin infusion** should be started.
  - Reversible causes of seizure activity (infection, electrolyte imbalance) should be treated.
    - If relevant, anticonvulsant levels should be measured.
    - Intravenous glucose or thiamine should be given if poor nutrition or alcoholism is suspected.
- A patient in status epilepticus for more than **30 minutes** should be transferred to the intensive therapy unit (ITU) and treated with **general anaesthesia** (e.g. propofol, barbiturates) for 12–24 hours after the last clinical/electrographic seizure. Ideally, EEG monitoring should be continuous.

16.3 EPILEPSY

DEFINITION

- Epilepsy is a predisposition to recurrent unprovoked seizures.

CLINICAL FEATURES

- See previous material regarding seizures.

MANAGEMENT

- **Non-pharmacological**:
  - Avoidance of activities that would be hazardous if a seizure were to occur (e.g. swimming, operating heavy machinery and driving).
- **Surgery**:
  - Surgery may be indicated in medically intractable epilepsy if a discrete epileptogenic zone can be identified and mapped using EEG.

Neurological disorders

Table 16.1 **Common anticonvulsant agents**

DRUG	INDICATION	SIDE EFFECTS
Carbamazepine	*First line* for focal seizures ± secondary generalisation	Rash; bone marrow suppression (rarely); liver enzyme inducer
Sodium valproate	*First line* for generalised seizures; focal seizures ± secondary generalisation	Acute liver damage; hair loss (hair regrows); weight gain; tremor (at high doses)
Phenytoin	Generalised tonic-clonic seizures; focal seizures	Hirsuitism, gum hypertrophy, rash; liver enzyme inducer **Toxicity**: nystagmus, drowsiness, confusion, cerebellar signs
Lamotrigine	*First line*: monotherapy or adjunct for generalised and focal seizures	Rash; may worsen myoclonus
Topiramate	Adjunct with other treatment for focal seizures	Sedation; nausea, weight loss, poor appetite; behavioural disturbance; liver enzyme inducer
Levetirecetam (Keppra®)	*Second line:* monotherapy or adjunct for focal seizures ± secondary generalisation	Asthenia; drowsiness; gastrointestinal disturbance; rash; behavioural disturbance

- Surgery has been particularly successful for control of unilateral temporal lobe epilepsy (often due to mesial temporal sclerosis).
- Vagus nerve stimulators can be effective in patients poorly controlled despite a good trial of more than two anti-epileptic drugs.
- **Pharmacological**:
  - Anticonvulsant therapy (see **Table 16.1**) is usually initiated after a patient suffers a second unprovoked seizure.
  - The dose should be titrated to control seizures and minimise side effects.
  - If one drug is unsuccessful, a second-line drug or an adjunct should be considered.

MICRO-print

Epilepsy in women of childbearing age

- Many anticonvulsant drugs (carbamazepine, phenytoin, phenobarbitone, primidone, topiramate) are hepatic enzyme inducing and may render the oral contraceptive pill ineffective; alternative contraception should be considered.

continued...

continued...

- Anticonvulsants in pregnancy:
  - If a woman with epilepsy becomes pregnant or is planning to become pregnant, anticonvulsant medication should be rationalised.
  - The potential teratogenicity risks and risk from uncontrolled seizures need to be discussed with the patient.
  - Valproate is contraindicated as a first-line therapy for idiopathic generalised epilepsy (IDE) in women of childbearing age because it has the highest risk of teratogenicity (major foetal malformations, including neural tube defects).
  - Ideally, a patient's symptoms should be well controlled prior to the pregnancy.
  - Patients may experience an increase, decrease or no change in seizure frequency during pregnancy.
  - Drug levels of levitarecetam and lamotrogine decrease significantly during pregnancy.
  - Folate supplementation is advised for all women planning to become pregnant to reduce the risk of neural tube defects.

16.4 NON-EPILEPTIC SEIZURES

- It is important to consider all potential differential diagnoses in a patient presenting with clinical features suggestive of a seizure. Non-epileptic seizure events are not related to abnormal electrical activity in the brain and should not receive anti-convulsant therapy.
- It is estimated that almost 20% of suspected seizures are actually non-epileptic seizures (may also occur in patients with epileptic seizures).
- There are numerous causes, the most common being cardiogenic (see the following MICRO-print).
- **Psychogenic non-epileptic seizures**:
  - These are due to an underlying psychological disorder.
  - They are more common in females, usually first occurring in the late teenage years or early adulthood.
  - Patients may have experienced traumatic life events in the past (often physical/sexual abuse).
  - They have a highly variable pattern and may resemble true seizures (although some features are suggestive: biting tip of tongue, gradual-onset seizure, eyes closed during seizures, seizure lasting longer than 2 minutes).
  - Significant injury is uncommon but can occur.
  - EEG recording during an event is normal.
- Management involves behavioural therapies and withdrawal of any anticonvulsant medication that may have been commenced.

Neurological disorders

MICRO-print

It is essential to consider cardiogenic collapse in all patients who experience transient loss of consciousness (T-LOC). All patients must have an electrocardiogram (ECG) to look for arrhythmias or long QT syndrome. If there is further suspicion of cardiac origin (family history of sudden death in early adulthood, symptoms during exercise, no aura, no focal onset), then further investigations include 24-hour ECG, echocardiogram and implantable cardiac recording devices (Reveal®).

MICRO-case

Generalised tonic-clonic seizures

A 13-year-old schoolgirl is bought to the emergency department after experiencing a 'seizure'. Approximately 15 minutes prior, she was playing on her dance mat when her father heard her fall to the floor. He rushed straight into the lounge where he found her apparently seizing. He describes rhythmic movements of her arms and legs. He also noticed that her eyes were 'rolled back in her head', her lips went blue, and she was unresponsive. The seizure lasted for approximately 1 minute. By the time the paramedics arrived, the seizure had stopped, but she remained confused and drowsy. As a younger child, she suffered from recurrent febrile seizures but is otherwise fit and well.

She has been well recently but has been upset since her grandmother passed away.

On examination, she appears drowsy, but her Glasgow Coma Scale (GCS) score is 15/15. Her trousers are wet, and she has bitten her tongue. She has a large bruise to her left jaw, and it looks very swollen. Otherwise, examination is normal, and she has no neurological deficit. An X-ray reveals a fractured jaw. A provisional diagnosis of generalised seizure is made.

She is given advice regarding risk avoidance and the implications of anticonvulsant therapy, especially on pregnancy, are discussed (should it need to be started in the future).

Summary points

- Generalised seizures commonly result in significant injuries, especially when patients do not experience a preceding aura, which can act as a warning.
- Education about epilepsy is imperative. Patients and their families should be informed about avoiding risky behaviour during which a seizure would be dangerous, such as bathing alone or driving. Information about anticonvulsant therapies and their side effects is also useful.
- Female patients will require additional counselling regarding the potential interactions between anticonvulsant therapy and pregnancy.

17 Headache and facial pain

17.1 OVERVIEW

- Headache is one of the most common neurological presenting complaints, and there are many causes. A detailed history is vital for an accurate diagnosis.
- It is important to differentiate benign **primary** headaches from potentially dangerous **secondary** causes that may require urgent investigation and management or even be imminently life threatening:
  - **primary headache**: headache occurring without an identifiable external cause (e.g. tension headache, migraine, cluster headache);
  - **secondary headache**: headache due to an underlying disease process, which may be suggested by the presence of **red flag symptoms** (see **Table 17.1**).

Table 17.1 Red flag features of headache

RED FLAG SYMPTOMS	SUGGESTIVE OF
Fever, meningism	Meningitis or encephalitis
Morning headache, papilloedema	Raised intracranial pressure
Focal neurological deficit	Space-occupying lesion (tumour, abscess)
Sudden onset 'thunderclap' headache	Subarachnoid haemorrhage, parenchymal haemorrhage
Scalp tenderness, jaw claudication	Temporal arteritis
Red eye, fixed dilated pupil	Acute closed-angle glaucoma

17.2 ACUTE-ONSET HEADACHE

> **MICRO-facts**
>
> Sudden-onset headache should always raise suspicion of **subarachnoid haemorrhage**. Early diagnosis and intervention, particularly of a small warning bleed from a berry aneurysm, may facilitate life-saving treatment.

- Important causes to consider (see **Table 17.1** for red flag features):
  - **intracranial haemorrhage** (subarachnoid haemorrhage/parenchymal haemorrhage): see Section 12.2;
  - **meningitis/encephalitis**: see Sections 12.1, 12.2, 19.1, 19.2;
  - **temporal arteritis** (giant cell arteritis): see Section 21.1.

SINUSITIS

- Inflammation of the mucous membranes of the paranasal sinuses (maxillary, frontal, ethmoid and sphenoid) causes obstruction and pooling of secretions.
- Inflammation is most commonly a result of infection but may also be related to an allergic reaction or autoimmune disease.
- Infection is usually viral but may be fungal or bacterial (30–40% of cases) (*Streptococcus pneumoniae, Haemophilus influenzae, Moraxella catarrhalis*).
- Dental infection is occasionally associated with maxillary sinusitis.

CLINICAL FEATURES

- Acute or chronic (symptoms for > 12 consecutive weeks). Acute sinusitis is usually a result of viral infection.
- Headache (frontal, often with facial pain that is worse on movement and tenderness over the involved sinuses).
- Purulent nasal discharge.
- Fever/systemic illness.
- Nasal obstruction.

INVESTIGATION

- Clinical diagnosis but computed tomographic (CT) imaging may help.

MANAGEMENT

- Simple analgesia.
- Intranasal decongestants useful for short-term relief but should not be used for longer than 7 days.
- Antibiotics only used when systemic infection present.
- Surgical drainage if refractory to medical treatment.

COMPLICATIONS

- Spread of infection in the orbit may produce orbital cellulitis or even cavernous sinus thrombosis.
- Intracranial spread may cause meningitis, encephalitis or an intracranial abscess.

17.3 ACUTE-ONSET RECURRENT HEADACHES

- Diagnosis of recurrent headache can clearly only be made after several episodes. More sinister causes of acute headache should always be considered on first presentation.

MIGRAINE

DEFINITION

- Migraine is classically described as a chronic unilateral throbbing headache that may or may not be associated with an aura.

EPIDEMIOLOGY

- **Gender**: more common in females (3:1).
- **Lifetime prevalence**: 12–28%.
- **Age**:
  - Peak age of onset in both sexes is middle age.
  - Before puberty, migraine is more common in boys than girls.
  - After menopause, the number of female sufferers declines so that prevalence is equal in both sexes.
- Approximately 70% of migraine sufferers have an affected first-degree relative. No genetic basis has yet been identified.

PATHOPHYSIOLOGY

- A primary neuronal hyperexcitability has been implicated with secondary changes in cerebral perfusion.
- A number of drugs used to treat migraine are vasoactive, whereas others have no detectable effect on cerebral perfusion.
- It is likely that migraine represents the common presentation of multiple as-yet-uncharacterised pathogenic mechanisms.

MIGRAINE TRIGGERS

- A number of different factors have been reported to trigger migraine attacks. An individual is likely to be aware of his or her own triggers:
  - emotional upset;
  - food: red wine, chocolate, cheese, monosodium glutamate, caffeine, tyramine;

Neurological disorders

- sensory stimulation: strobe lighting, smells, loud noises, extremes of heat/cold;
- drugs: vasodilators;
- sleep disturbance;
- hormonal change: menstruation, oral contraceptive pill/hormone replacement therapy, menopause.

CLINICAL FEATURES

- **Headache**
  - Headache is variable, but typically unilateral, focused around the frontotemporal or ocular area and throbbing in nature.
  - Onset is usually subacute and duration is 4–72 hours.
  - There are non-specific associated symptoms such as nausea, vomiting and reduced appetite.
  - Photophobia or phonophobia may be present.
- **Aura**
  - The aura consists of transient neurological symptoms, which may accompany or precede the headache. Typically, it lasts approximately 20 minutes.
  - Aura can occur in isolation without headache (acephalgic migraine).
  - Described auras include the following:
    - **visual symptoms**:
      - commonly a scintillating scotoma, an area of absent vision surrounded by a shimmering border, which migrates across the visual field;
      - negative visual auras, including field defects and complete blindness.
    - **paraesthesia**:
      - second most common aura after visual;
      - sensory disturbance positive or negative; often a positive phenomenon (tingling) is followed by numbness.
    - **weakness**: most commonly described as limb heaviness, often without objectively detectable weakness (distinct from a hemiplegic migraine).
  - **Migraine variants**: The headache is less prominent than another manifestation:
    - **Hemiplegic migraine**:
      - This is a rare migraine syndrome featuring temporary hemiparesis with or without sensory disturbance.
      - Headache does occur but is usually less dramatic than the neurological deficit.
      - The weakness is more persistent and usually more severe than a motor aura.

- **Abdominal migraine**:
  - ○ This form of migraine is more common in younger patients.
  - ○ The prominent symptom is abdominal pain rather than headache.
  - ○ Often, as the patient matures into adulthood, a more typical migraine syndrome develops.

INVESTIGATIONS

- Clinical diagnosis.
- New-onset migraine with associated focal neurological deficit requires investigation to exclude another underlying condition.

MANAGEMENT

- **Abortive therapy** for an acute attack:
  - **First line**: Treatment is with simple analgesia (paracetamol, high-dose aspirin [900 mg], ibuprofen). Use of an antiemetic may be beneficial.
  - **Second line**: Treatment is with a $5HT_1$ (serotonin) agonist such as sumatriptan:
    - often given as a subcutaneous injection due to superior bioavailability and speed of onset;
    - produces vasoconstriction and therefore contraindicated in patients with a history of myocardial infarction.
- **Prophylaxis**:
  - Indicated when migraine attacks are particularly frequent or disabling;
  - **First line**: beta-blocker (propranolol); tricyclic antidepressant (e.g. amitriptyline); or pizotifen (a serotonin antagonist);
  - **Second line**: sodium valproate, verapamil, topiramate.

PROGNOSIS

- Most patients respond well to treatment, and many experience remission with increasing age.
- Very occasionally, a migraine may be associated with permanent neurological deficit.
- There is a slight increased risk of stroke in migraine sufferers; patients with other modifiable risk factors should be counselled on the absolute risk of stroke.

CLUSTER HEADACHE

DEFINITION

- Cluster headaches are severe unilateral periorbital headaches that often occur in clusters and are associated with autonomic features.

PATHOPHYSIOLOGY

- These headaches are poorly understood, but thought to be a neurovascular phenomenon.
- The clustering of attacks has implicated involvement of the hypothalamus.
- Disinhibition of nociceptive and autonomic pathways has also been suggested.

EPIDEMIOLOGY

- **Prevalence**: approximately 124 per 100,000.
- **Gender**: more common in men (5:1).
- **Age**: onset normally between the ages of 30 and 50 years.
- Positive family history in about 10%.

CLINICAL FEATURES

- **Headache**: typically unilateral periorbital pain with a relatively short duration (up to 3 hours); classically occurs at the same time each day, often at the onset of REM (rapid eye movement) sleep.
- **Autonomic symptoms**: often associated with the headache, including lacrimation, conjunctival injection, rhinorrhoea, perspiration and an ipsilateral Horner's syndrome.
- Attacks occur in clusters consisting of one to two attacks per day for 4–12 weeks.
- Patients may describe specific triggers for attacks, including drugs (e.g. glyceryltrinitrate (GTN) spray), foods, alcohol and smoking.

INVESTIGATIONS

- Clinical diagnosis, but investigation is recommended for a first episode to rule out alternative causes of focal neurological deficit.

MANAGEMENT

- Specialist neurological opinion advised.
- **Abortive therapy**:
  - Cluster headaches do not respond to simple analgesia.
  - High-flow oxygen for 20 minutes may abort an attack.
  - Subcutaneous sumatriptan can be used.
- **Prophylaxis**: verapamil.

PROGNOSIS

- There is no definitive cure; most patients eventually experience remission.

> **MICRO-print**
> **Chronic paroxysmal hemicrania**
> Chronic paroxysmal hemicrania (CPH) consists of a group of disorders, which are similar to cluster headache but with shorter-duration attacks that may occur 2–40 times per day and in a less-predictable manner. All of these disorders respond to indomethacin treatment.

TRIGEMINAL NEURALGIA

DEFINITION

- Trigeminal neuralgia is a hemifacial pain syndrome associated with the distribution of the trigeminal nerve; it may be accompanied by facial spasm.

PATHOPHYSIOLOGY

- Usually unknown but can be due to irritation by a structural lesion such as an overlying blood vessel or multiple sclerosis (MS) plaque.

EPIDEMIOLOGY

- **Age**: more common in patients aged older than 50 years.
- **Gender**: more common in females (3:2).

CLINICAL FEATURES

- Electric shock-like pain occurs in trigeminal nerve distribution, almost always unilaterally (more commonly affects the right side of the face).
  - Pain lasts for seconds only and is provoked by movement, eating, changes in temperature and sensory stimulation of the area.
  - The pattern of attacks is highly variable: Patients may suffer one or hundreds of attacks per day, lasting for days or months.
- It is not associated with any other neurological deficit.

INVESTIGATIONS

- Clinical diagnosis.
- **Magnetic resonance imaging (MRI) of the brain**: may be useful to discover a secondary cause of trigeminal nerve irritation and should be performed in all patients younger than 50 years.

MANAGEMENT

- Anticonvulsant drugs, especially carbamazepine.
- Muscle relaxants (e.g. baclofen).

Neurological disorders

- A secondary structural lesion may require surgical intervention. Microvascular decompression of an overlying blood vessel can be curative.
- Radiosurgery with a gamma knife can be performed if co-morbidities preclude surgery.

PROGNOSIS

- Patients usually respond to anticonvulsant therapy. Spontaneous remission may occur.

> **MICRO-facts**
>
> An important differential diagnosis for trigeminal neuralgia is temporal arteritis (especially since eating can trigger an attack). Blood inflammatory markers are usually normal in trigeminal neuralgia but almost always elevated in temporal arteritis.

GLAUCOMA

- Glaucoma is caused by raised intraocular pressure. Onset of primary open-angle glaucoma is chronic; however, acute closed-angle glaucoma, which requires emergency treatment, presents acutely.
- Both forms may present with headache, particularly ipsilateral periorbital pain. Other important symptoms to identify include red eye, visual 'halos' and history of ocular disease.
- Patients do not always report visual loss because the central visual field is affected very late in the disease.
- In acute closed-angle glaucoma, the pupil may be fixed and dilated.
- Diagnosis is based on history and examination.
- Acute closed-angle glaucoma requires urgent management to avoid visual loss.
    - First-line treatment is with intravenous acetazolamide, a topical beta-blocker and a topical steroid.
    - Urgent ophthalmology input is required; surgical options include laser iridotomy.

17.4 CHRONIC HEADACHES

TENSION HEADACHE

DEFINITION

- Tension is the most common cause of headache, accounting for about 90% of all headaches.
- The pathogenesis is not well understood, but by definition the condition is benign.

- Pain is thought to be related to abnormal tension in muscles of the neck and scalp; notable precipitating factors include stress, tiredness, dehydration and poor posture.
- Chronic tension headache is defined as occurring on more than 15 days/month for at least 6 months.

EPIDEMIOLOGY

- **Prevalence**: Around half the general adult population suffer from occasional tension headaches, and approximately 3% suffer from chronic tension headaches.

CLINICAL FEATURES

- Patients usually describe a 'tight band' around the head:
    - mild-to-moderate intensity;
    - usually bilateral;
    - usually in isolation rather than in combination with other symptoms;
    - onset usually subacute.

INVESTIGATIONS

- Clinical diagnosis. If atypical features are present, other causes of headache should be excluded.

MANAGEMENT

- Reassurance that the prognosis is benign. Patients should be advised to avoid precipitating factors if possible.
- **Analgesia**: should be used with caution as chronic use can result in **analgesia overuse headache** (see next MICRO-print).
    - For occasional tension headache, treatment with simple analgesia such as paracetamol and ibuprofen is appropriate.
    - For chronic tension headache, consideration should be given to a preventive treatment such as amitriptyline.

MICRO-print

Analgesic overuse headache

Frequent analgesic use may cause a chronic daily headache (e.g. codeine, often prescribed for the treatment of headaches, may, if overused, result in analgesic overuse headache).

- Treatment is by withdrawal of the analgesia, which may initially cause a worsening in symptoms.
- Alternative treatment should be considered for the primary condition (e.g. prophylaxis in migraine).

Neurological disorders

RAISED INTRACRANIAL PRESSURE

DEFINITION

- Pathologically raised pressure inside of the cranial cavity can be caused by increased volume of blood, cerebrospinal fluid (CSF) or parenchymal tissue (see Sections 5.2, 12.1 and 12.2; and Chapters 13 and 19).

AETIOLOGY

- **Hydrocephalus.**
- **Space-occupying lesion**:
  - **tumour**: primary or metastatic (most common cause);
  - brain abscess or other infective lesions (e.g. toxoplasmosis or tuberculoma).
- **Cerebral oedema**: can occur as a result of meningitis/encephalitis, acute liver failure, hypertensive encephalopathy, hypercapnia or rapid osmotic shifts.
- **Intracranial haemorrhage**:
  - Most often this is as a result of an arterial bleed (extradural haemorrhage, subarachnoid haemorrhage); subsequent oedema will lead to further rise in intracranial pressure.
  - A venous bleed (subdural haemorrhage) or venous outflow obstruction (e.g. venous sinus thrombosis) may also cause raised intracranial pressure.

CLINICAL FEATURES

- **Headache**: typically described as 'throbbing' and worse on waking from sleep and when straining, coughing, etc.
- Papilloedema (usually bilateral but occasionally unilateral).
- Drowsiness.
- Vomiting.
- Abducens nerve (VI) palsy (false localising sign).
- **Cushing's triad**: hypertension, bradycardia and disrupted ventilation occurring as a result of increased intracranial pressure – warning sign of imminent brain herniation.
- Seizures.

INVESTIGATIONS

- **Brain imaging**:
  - **CT/MRI Brain**: may allow rapid identification of a lesion, particularly an acute haemorrhage. Mass effect and midline shift may be visible.

- A contrast scan is necessary to exclude a space-occupying lesion such as a malignancy.
- **CT/magnetic resonance venography**: Identification of a venous sinus thrombosis may be made this way.
- Lumbar puncture is **contraindicated** in patients with features of raised intracranial pressure until imaging has ruled out obstructive hydrocephalus (should be discussed with neurosurgeons).

MANAGEMENT AND PROGNOSIS

- Dependent on the underlying cause.
- Severe raised intracranial pressure may result in fatal herniation of the brain through its supporting structures and even the foramen magnum (coning).

MICRO-print

Idiopathic intracranial hypertension

- Idiopathic intracranial hypertension (IIH) is raised CSF pressure in the absence of another identified cause.
- It is assumed to be a communicating hydrocephalus produced by reduced absorption of CSF, but pathophysiology remains unclear.
- **Clinical presentation:**
  - Typically, it occurs in young, obese women.
  - It is present with features of raised intracranial pressure.
  - Lumbar puncture reveals a high opening pressure (typically > 40 cm H_2O).
  - It is important to identify papilloedema if present and any history of visual disturbance; untreated IIH may be sight threatening.
- Venous sinus thrombosis is an important differential diagnosis (especially if patient is using oestrogen-containing contraception).
- **Management:**
  - **Weight loss** alone is effective treatment for IIH.
  - **Carbonic anhydrase inhibitors:** Acetazolamide is the first-line treatment.
  - **Surgery:**
    - Intermittent lumbar puncture will relieve the raised intracranial pressure, but a ventriculoperitoneal or lumboperitoneal shunt is more effective.
    - Optic nerve fenestration is used if sight is threatened.

Neurological disorders

MICRO-case

Migraine

A 24-year-old woman presents to her general practitioner (GP) with headaches. They have been occurring frequently over the past few months and are starting to interfere with her work.

They are always on the right side of her head and are gradual in onset, normally starting midmorning. Before each headache, she describes 'zigzag' lines in her vision, and once the headache starts, she cannot tolerate the light, feels sick and often vomits. She has had to leave work early on occasion, and her seniors are increasingly concerned.

On further questioning, she has no symptoms of raised intracranial pressure, and there are no obvious precipitating factors for her headaches, although she has mentioned that she has been drinking more coffee recently. Paracetamol and ibuprofen have been tried but have provided little relief.

On examination, she has no focal neurological deficit; her cardiovascular, respiratory and gastrointestinal examinations are normal.

The diagnosis of migraine is made, and she is advised regarding appropriate analgesia and avoidance of triggers such as caffeine.

She sees her GP after 3 months for a review, and her headaches are much improved.

Summary points

- Recurrent headaches can be very disabling and have significant effects on both work and personal relationships.
- There are many possible triggers for migraines; thus, taking a thorough history is vital.
- Multiple treatments are available for migraine; therefore, if one fails to work, others should be tried.

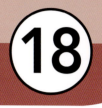

Neurocutaneous disorders

18.1 OVERVIEW

- Neurocutaneous disorders are a collection of hereditary disorders characterized by neurological and skin abnormalities.
- Much of the pathology is associated with the development of tumours of neural tissues.

18.2 NEUROFIBROMATOSIS

DEFINITION

- Neurofibromatosis disorders are associated with the formation of neurofibromas (benign Schwann cell tumours):
    - neurofibromatosis type 1 (NF1): predominantly cutaneous features;
    - neurofibromatosis type 2 (NF2): predominantly central nervous system (CNS) tumours.

NEUROFIBROMATOSIS TYPE 1 (VON RECKLINGHAUSEN'S DISEASE)

EPIDEMIOLOGY

- **Incidence**: approximately 1 in 3000 live births.
- **Gender**: males = females.
- **Age**: NF1 usually becomes clinically apparent in late childhood or early adolescence with the development of cutaneous features.

AETIOLOGY

- NF1 is an autosomal dominant disorder due to mutation or deletion in the NF1 gene on chromosome 17.
- The gene product neurofibromin is thought to be a tumour suppressor.

CLINICAL FEATURES

- **Cutaneous**:
  - **Neurofibromas**: These are actually neural tumours.
  - **Café-au-lait spots**: These are light brown patches on the trunk with well-demarcated edges; they may be present at birth or appear over time.
  - **Axillary or inguinal freckles** are present.
- **Ocular**:
  - **Lisch nodules**: small, melanocytic iris hamartomas seen on slit-lamp examination in 90% of affected patients over the age of 10 years;
  - **Optic gliomas**: occur in about 15% of patients with NF1; may cause visual impairment if untreated.
- **Skeletal dysplasia**:
  - Scoliosis;
  - Sphenoid wing dysplasia, which can cause exopthalmos;
  - Short stature;
  - Tibial pseudoarthrosis;
  - Macrocephaly.
- **Neurological**: Various neurological tumours are associated with NF1 and affect both the CNS and more commonly the peripheral nervous system (PNS) (may undergo malignant transformation). Included are meningioma, vestibular schwannoma, glioma and neurofibroma.
  - **Neurofibromas**:
    - These develop from fibrous tissue surrounding the peripheral nerve sheath.
    - They cannot be surgically separated from the nerve without disrupting function (unlike schwannomas).
    - Since they affect peripheral nerves, neurofibromas are often apparent on superficial examination.
    - **Plexiform neurofibromas**: These affect proximal nerves and may be locally invasive.
    - **Subcutaneous neurofibromas**: These affect nerves more distally with subcutaneous swellings associated with altered sensation in the distribution of the affected sensory nerve.
    - **Mollusca fibrosa**: The most peripheral nerves are affected; mollusca fibrosa presents as painless, pedunculated, purplish lesions.
  - NF1 is associated with the development of cognitive and learning disability in a small proportion of affected individuals.
- **Endocrine**: NF1 is associated with multiple endocrine neoplasia (MEN) syndromes; common tumours include phaeochromocytoma and medullary carcinoma of the thyroid.

> **MICRO-print**
>
> **Diagnostic criteria for neurofibromatosis type 1**
>
> Diagnosis of NF1 is made if two or more of the following are present:
>
> - six or more café-au-lait spots: larger than 5 mm before puberty, larger than 15 mm after puberty;
> - two or more neurofibromas of any type or one plexiform;
> - axillary or inguinal freckles;
> - optic glioma;
> - two or more Lisch nodules;
> - first-degree relative with NF1;
> - sphenoid dysplasia.

INVESTIGATIONS

- **Imaging**: Magnetic resonance imaging (MRI) is used for detection of intracranial tumours and optic gliomas. Plain radiographs may reveal skeletal abnormalities.
- **Slit-lamp examination**: This is used for detection of Lisch nodules and is helpful in assessing the likelihood of NF1 if there is a positive family history.
- **Genetic testing**: Screening for mutations of the NF1 gene has about 95% sensitivity.
- Urinary and plasma catecholamines are used to screen for phaeochromocytoma.

MANAGEMENT

- Best managed by a diverse multidisciplinary team (MDT).
- No cure; treatment is focused on ameliorating specific complications if and when they arise:
  - Symptomatic tumours, particularly intracranial tumours, may require excision or radiotherapy.
  - Skeletal abnormalities such as scoliosis may also require specific surgical treatment.
- Genetic counselling is important.

PROGNOSIS

- On average, NF1 reduces life expectancy by 15 years.

NEUROFIBROMATOSIS TYPE 2

EPIDEMIOLOGY

- **Incidence**: estimated about 1 in 25,000 live births.
- **Age**: usually becomes clinically apparent in young adults aged 15–25 years.

Neurological disorders

Aetiology

- NF2 is an autosomal dominant condition due to mutation or deletion in the NF2 gene on chromosome 22.
- Like neurofibromin, the NF2 gene product merlin is a tumour suppressor. Unlike NF1, 50% of NF2 cases arise from a new mutation (sporadic cases).

Clinical features

- Cutaneous features are unusual in NF2.
- Subcutaneous masses do occur, but these tend to be schwannomas rather than neurofibromas as in NF1.
- CNS tumours are typical of NF2, but malignant transformation is less common than in NF1.
  - NF2 often presents with sensorineural hearing loss due to bilateral vestibular schwannomas.
  - Optic gliomas can occur in NF2, but Lisch nodules are not commonly seen. Patients often develop juvenile cataracts.

MICRO-print

Diagnostic criteria for neurofibromatosis type 2

To be diagnosed with NF2, a patient must fulfill one of the following criteria:

- bilateral VIII nerve tumours on MRI brain;
- unilateral VIII nerve tumour on MRI brain and a first-degree relative with NF2;
- first-degree relative with NF2 and two of meningioma, glioma, schwannoma and juvenile cataracts.

Investigation and management

- Investigation and management are the same as for NF1.
- No cure is available; focus is on detection and management of complications, particularly intracranial tumours.
  - Audiometry and brainstem evoked potentials may be useful in detecting vestibular schwannomas before they are apparent on imaging.
  - Genetic testing is less sensitive than in NF1; a mutation is only detectable in approximately 65% of cases.

Prognosis

- Like NF1, prognosis in NF2 is variable depending on the number and distribution of tumours, but life expectancy is usually less than with NF1.

MICRO-print

Vestibular schwannoma (acoustic neuroma)

- Benign tumour of the Schwann cells along the vestibulocochlear nerve (VIII) between the cerebellopontine angle and the internal auditory meatus in the petrous temporal bone.
- Diagnosis should prompt consideration of neurofibromatosis.
- Clinical features:
    - There is ipsilateral sensorineural hearing loss, tinnitus, vertigo and an ipsilateral trigeminal nerve palsy.
    - Larger tumours may also involve the facial nerve to produce an ipsilateral lower motor neuron facial nerve palsy and lead to raised ICP.
- MRI brain is usually diagnostic; formal audiometry may be used to objectively identify and characterise hearing loss.
- Conservative management with annual MRI surveillance may be appropriate for smaller tumours.
- Surgical resection is employed in larger tumours.
- Radiotherapy is used if surgery is not possible.

18.3 TUBEROUS SCLEROSIS

DEFINITION

- Tuberous sclerosis is a multisystem disorder associated with hamartoma formation in various organ systems.

EPIDEMIOLOGY

- **Prevalence**: estimated to occur in approximately 1 in 6000 live births.
- **Gender**: males = females.
- **Age**: may present at any age but neurological involvement usually presents in childhood.

AETIOLOGY

- There is autosomal dominant inheritance related to mutations in the tuberous sclerosis gene 1 (TSC1) on chromosome 9 (encoding hamartin) and the tuberous sclerosis gene 2 (TSC2) on chromosome 16 (encoding tuberin).
- Both of these gene products are thought to be tumour suppressors.
- Two-thirds of cases occur sporadically due to *de novo* mutations.

CLINICAL FEATURES

- **Skin**:
  - **Ash leaf macules**: areas of depigmentation, usually multiple, commonly found on trunk (seen using a Wood's lamp);
  - **Shagreen patches**: irregular thick plaques on sacrum and back with orange peel or leathery texture;
  - **Periungal fibroma**: smooth, firm, flesh-coloured growths adjacent to or rising under nails;
  - **Confetti lesions**: cluster of hypopigmented lesions, reticulated appearance; can appear anywhere on skin.
- **Neurological**:
  - **Epilepsy**: initially focal but may become generalised;
  - **Subependymal nodules**: small lesions occurring in the walls of the cerebral ventricles; do not enlarge or cause hydrocephalus;
  - **Subependymal giant cell astrocytomas**: arise close to ventricles and may cause obstructive hydrocephalus;
  - Developmental delay and learning difficulties.
- **Renal**:
  - **Renal angiomyolipoma**: a benign hamartoma of the kidney that occurs in 50–80% of patients.
  - **Renal cell carcinoma**: affects less than 1% of patients.
  - **Tuberous sclerosis**: also a cause of polycystic kidney disease.
- **Cardiac**:
  - **Rhabdomyomas** occur in young children. Most spontaneously regress but should be monitored as they may enlarge and cause symptoms in puberty (e.g. arrhythmias, heart failure).
- **Pulmonary**:
  - Multifocal micronodular pneumocyte hyperplasia occurs in 50% of patients. It is usually asymptomatic but may be apparent as multiple nodules visible on chest X-ray.
- **Ocular**:
  - Retinal harmartoma or astrocytoma.

MICRO-print

Diagnostic criteria for tuberous sclerosis

- Definite tuberous sclerosis: two major or one major plus two minor criteria.
- Probable tuberous sclerosis: one major plus one minor criterion.
- Possible tuberous sclerosis: one major or two minor features.

continued...

continued...

MAJOR	MINOR
Cardiac rhabdomyoma	Multiple pits in dental enamel
Cortical tuber	Hamartomatous rectal polyps
Facial angiofibroma	Bone cysts
Hypomelanotic macule (ash leaf spot) (≥3)	Radial migration lines in cerebral white matter
Lymphangiomyomatosis	Gingival fibromas
Renal angiomyolipoma	Retinal achromatic patches
Retinal hamartomas	Confetti skin lesions
Shagreen patch	Multiple renal cysts
Subependymal giant cell tumour	
Subependymal nodule	
Ungual or periungual fibromas	

MANAGEMENT

- As with neurofibromatosis, there is no cure for tuberous sclerosis, and the aim is amelioration of symptoms.
  - Tumours may be surgically removed if appropriate.
  - Seizures may be controlled by anticonvulsant medication.
- Genetic counselling should be provided.

PROGNOSIS

- Prognosis is hugely variable depending on the pattern of symptoms. Intractable epilepsy and renal failure are common causes of mortality.

18.4 STURGE–WEBER SYNDROME

DEFINITION

- Sturge–Weber syndrome is a neurocutaneous disorder characterised by congenital hamartomatous malformations that affect the eye, skin and CNS.

EPIDEMIOLOGY

- **Prevalence**: about 1 in 50,000 live births.
- **Gender**: males = females.

Aetiology

- No genetic basis has yet been identified.
- Thought to result from failure of regression of the embryonic vascular plexus producing angiomata of related tissues.
- Neurological dysfunction occurs due to secondary effects on the surrounding brain tissue, including hypoxia, venous occlusion and thrombosis.

Clinical features

- Capillary naevus or 'port-wine stain' affecting one side of a patient's face is present from birth. It usually involves the forehead and upper eyelid in the distribution of the first or first and second divisions of the trigeminal nerve.
- **Eye disorders**: These include buphthalmos (congenital glaucoma) and choroidal angioma. Patients are vulnerable to glaucoma, which should be identified and treated early to avoid irreversible damage.
- **Epilepsy**: Focal seizures usually appear during the first year of life on the contralateral side to the capillary naevus.
- Developmental delay is variable depending on the extent of neurological involvement.
- **Headaches**: These occur in 30–45% of children, often as migraine-like episodes due to vascular disease.

Investigations

- **Imaging**:
  - Angiography allows identification of vascular abnormalities.
  - Skull X-ray can reveal characteristic parallel linear cortical calcification (tram-line sign).
- A complete ophthalmologic evaluation is necessary to identify glaucoma if present.

Management

- Seizures may be controlled with anticonvulsants. Intractable seizures may benefit from resection of an epileptic focus.
- Cosmetic camouflage creams can help conceal a capillary naevus, or it can be removed with laser therapy.
- Glaucoma should be managed aggressively.

Prognosis

- Most infants with Sturge–Weber syndrome develop seizures during the first year of life, and more than 50% of cases have severe learning difficulties by late childhood.

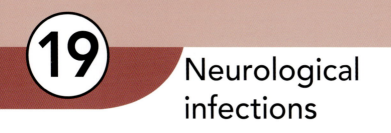

19 Neurological infections

19.1 MENINGITIS

DEFINITION

- Meningitis is an inflammation of the meninges, most commonly due to infection.

AETIOLOGY

- **Infection**: Bacterial, viral, or fungal.
- **Chemical**: Certain drugs and other substances can induce inflammation of the meninges.
- **Malignant**: Either direct spread or metastatic process.

CLINICAL FEATURES

- **Meningism**: headache, photophobia and neck stiffness (elicited on passive neck flexion):
  - Kernig's sign: Flexion of the hip joint with simultaneous knee extension produces shooting pain down the leg as a result of inflammation of the meninges surrounding the lumbar nerve roots.
  - Brudzinski's sign: There is involuntary flexion of the hips and knees when the neck is flexed.
- Fever.
- Systemic bacterial infection will produce signs of sepsis, including the purpuric rash associated with meningococcal sepsis.

BACTERIAL MENINGITIS

- Acute meningitis (<1 day) is almost always caused by a bacterial infection (see **Table 19.1**).

DIAGNOSIS

- **Lumbar puncture** (LP) and cerebrospinal fluid (CSF) examination (see **Table 19.2**):
  - Microscopy, culture and sensitivities. Separate samples should be used for prolonged tuberculosis (TB) and fungal culture if appropriate.
  - Serology: for antibodies against fungi and viruses.

- Differential white cell count and red cell count.
- Protein and glucose concentration.
- Polymerase chain reaction (PCR) for meningococcus, pneumococcus and viruses (includes enterovirus, mumps, varicella zoster virus [VZV], cytomegalovirus [CMV] and herpes simplex virus [HSV]).

Table 19.1 Bacterial causes of meningitis

ORGANISM	MICROSCOPIC APPEARANCE	OTHER FEATURES
Streptococcus pneumoniae	Gram-positive diplococci, may grow in chains	• Most common cause of bacterial meningitis
Neisseria meningitidis	Gram-negative intracellular diplococci	• Associated with crowding such as student dorms and military barracks. • Meningococcal septicaemia associated with non-blanching petechial rash. • Particularly common in the young.
Haemophilus influenzae	Gram-negative bacillus	• Isolation of *H. influenzae* suggests underlying URTI, immunosuppression or CSF leak. • More common in children/young adults. • Incidence has declined since the introduction of vaccination.
Staphylococcus aureus	Gram-positive cocci which form in clusters	• Important iatrogenic infection and in IVDU.
Listeria monocytogenes	Gram-positive bacillus	• Highest mortality. • Requires cover with amoxicillin in at-risk groups. • Important cause in very young and elderly
Mycobacterium tuberculosis	Acid-fast bacillus	• Subacute or chronic presentation. • Associated with immunosuppression.

Table 19.2 CSF examination in meningitis

CAUSE OF MENINGITIS	CELL COUNT AND DIFFERENTIAL	PROTEIN	GLUCOSE	MICROSCOPY/CYTOLOGY
Acute bacterial	Raised white count (>300mm^3)/ Neutrophils	Raised	Reduced	Organisms seen
Viral	Raised white cell count (<300mm^3) /Lymphocytes	Normal or raised	Normal	No organisms seen
Tuberculosis	Raised white cell count (<300mm^3)/ Mixed cell type or lymphocytes	Very raised	Reduced	Often no organisms seen. Fluorescence microscopy should be performed.
Fungal	Raised white cell count (<300mm^3)	Raised	Reduced	Often no organisms seen
Malignant	Raised white cell count /Neutrophils	Raised	Reduced	Atypical cells on cytology

- **Other microbiological specimens**:
  - blood cultures;
  - blood for meningococcal and pneumococcal PCR;
  - stool for enterovirus PCR.
- **Computed tomography (CT) of the head**:
  - required prior to LP to rule out an obstructive hydrocephalus if features of raised intracranial pressure (ICP) are present;
  - may show leptomeningeal enhancement in chronic meningitis (such as tuberculous meningitis).

MANAGEMENT

- **Antibiotics**: given as soon as possible.
  - **Community**: benzylpenicillin 1.2 g intramuscularly (IM) and immediate transfer to hospital.
  - **Hospital**:
    - Give cefotaxime 2 g intravenously (IV) immediately then continue QDS.
    - Do **not** delay for imaging/LP if there is a strong clinical suspicion of bacterial meningitis.

  – Ampicillin/amoxicillin are required to cover *Listeria monocytogenes* in those under 3 months or over 55 years old (if *Listeria* spp. are isolated, gentamicin should also be added).
  – **β-Lactam allergy**:
    ○ consult microbiologist;
    ○ chloramphenicol with vancomycin;
    ○ co-trimoxazole used to cover *Listeria*.
- Use of corticosteroids (dexamethasone) is controversial; benefit has been demonstrated in some studies, particularly with pneumococcal meningitis.
- **Contact tracing and prophylaxis**:
  - Rifampicin or ciprofloxacin may be required for close contact prophylaxis.
  - Effective vaccination for *Neisseria meningitidis* is available for serogroups A, C, Y and W135 and *Haemophilus influenzae* serotype B.
- **Supportive therapy**:
  - Make early contact with intensive care unit if patient is unstable.
  - The patient may require repeated CSF drainage if raised ICP is a significant problem.

COMPLICATIONS

- Cranial nerve palsies, including deafness due to vestibulocochlear nerve damage.
- Seizures.
- Focal neurological deficit such as hemiparesis.

PROGNOSIS

- Mortality in adult bacterial meningitis is approximately 20%.
- *Streptococcus pneumoniae* infection is associated with a worse prognosis than *N. meningitidis*.

VIRAL MENINGITIS

- Viruses are the most common cause of meningitis and produce less-severe disease than the bacterial form.

AETIOLOGY

- Enteroviruses (Coxsackie virus, echovirus, etc.).
- Mumps virus.
- HSV (usually HSV 2).
- Varicella zoster virus (VZV).
- Epstein–Barr virus (EBV).
- Cytomegalovirus (CMV).

CLINICAL FEATURES

- Clinical features are the same as for bacterial meningitis, although generally less severe and without systemic illness.

DIAGNOSIS

- As for bacterial meningitis.

MANAGEMENT

- Generally, only supportive treatment is necessary in immunocompetent individuals.
- HSV: acyclovir.
- CMV: ganciclovir.

TUBERCULOUS MENINGITIS

AETIOLOGY

- Tuberculous meningitis usually results from reactivation of latent *Mycobacteria tuberculosis* but can be due to a primary infection.

CLINICAL FEATURES

- Subacute onset of symptoms of meningitis (over weeks to months).
- Focal neurological deficit including isolated cranial nerve palsies.
- Weight loss.
- High-risk groups include:
    - those who are immunosuppressed, especially with HIV;
    - homeless;
    - alcoholics or intravenous drug users (IVDUs);
    - patients originating from prevalent areas (notably Africa and Asia).

DIAGNOSIS

- Diagnosis is the same as for bacterial meningitis.
- Fluorescence microscopy (auramine-rhodamine staining) should be performed on CSF, and TB PCR can be helpful.
- Definitive testing is by TB culture, which takes several weeks; if tuberculous meningitis is suspected, then cultures should not delay the initiation of treatment.

MANAGEMENT

- **Anti-TB agents** (usually for 12 months).
    - **Induction phase**: rifampicin, isoniazid, pyrazinamide and ethambutol for 2 months.
    - **Maintenance phase**: rifampicin and isoniazid for a further 10 months.
- Adjuvant steroids reduce mortality.
- Patients can deteriorate and develop tuberculomas even on appropriate treatment. Hydrocephalus due to basal meningeal inflammation can complicate the disease course; this is managed by serial LPs or a CSF shunting procedure.

Neurological disorders

Prognosis

- Mortality is approximately a third, even with appropriate therapy.

FUNGAL MENINGITIS

Aetiology

- Fungal meningitis is often associated with immunosuppressed states, such as in HIV:
  - *Cryptococcus neoformans* is the most common cause.
  - In immunocompetent or immunosuppressed patients, infection with *Histoplasma* spp., *Blastomyces* spp. or *Coccidiodes* spp. may occur (specific geographical distributions).
  - *Candida albicans* meningitis occurs in neonates and those with CSF shunts.

Diagnosis

- **CSF examination**: Staining with India ink shows presence of yeast in cryptococcal meningitis.
- Opening pressures are often very high and require regular LPs to maintain normal ICP.
- **Serology**: Cryptococcal antigen (CRAg) is detected in almost all cases of cryptococcal infection. Other serological tests are available.
- **CT head**: normal in 50% of cases. Mass lesions sometimes are seen.
- Fungal culture should not delay treatment if fungal meningitis is suspected.
- MRI may demonstrate lesions not visible on CT.

Management

- Amphotericin B is effective for the majority of fungi that can cause meningitis.
- Cryptococcal meningitis is almost always associated with very high ICPs, and daily LP or a temporary CSF shunt may be required.
- Lifelong fluconazole prophylaxis is required following cryptococcal meningitis in those who are immunosuppressed (or until immune restitution in HIV patients on HARRT).

MICRO-case

Bacterial meningitis

Baby Matthew is a preterm infant (born at 28 weeks) and is 4 hours old. The nurses on the neonatal ward alert the junior doctor that he is unwell and has a high temperature.

On examination, he is floppy and unresponsive, with a temperature of 39°C. He also appears jaundiced. *continued…*

continued…

Meningitis is suspected and empirical antimicrobial therapy is commenced, including intravenous cefotaxime, amoxicillin and aciclovir given immediately. Blood samples are taken for full blood count, U&Es, liver function tests (LFTs) and cultures. A urine sample is sent, a LP performed and a chest X-ray requested.

The CSF appeared cloudy, with increased polymorphs and protein and reduced glucose. The blood culture results were negative, and the urine sample and X-ray showed no evidence of infection.

Baby Matthew remained on the neonatal intensive care unit for several weeks but recovered. He was, however, found to be profoundly deaf as a result of his meningitis.

Summary points

- Presentation of sepsis in neonates is non-specific, and cultures should be taken from as many sites as possible to confirm a diagnosis.
- Blood cultures are often negative when taken after administration of antibiotics and should not be relied on solely.
- Common organisms in neonates are bacteria that colonise the birth canal. These include group B *Streptococcus, Listeria monocytogenes* and *Escherichia coli.*
- Viral PCR for HSV, VZV and enteroviruses along with meningococcal and pneumococcal PCRs are performed routinely on CSF samples.
- Penicillin or a third-generation cephalosporin should be administered as soon as there is a suspicion of meningitis.
- There are many potential complications for children who survive meningitis, of which hearing loss and neurodevelopmental delay are two examples.

19.2 ENCEPHALITIS

Definition

- Encephalitis is an inflammation of the brain parenchyma.

Aetiology

- HSV (usually HSV1) is the most common cause of encephalitis.
- Arboviruses: Tick-borne encephalitis, Japanese B encephalitis virus, West Nile virus, equine encephalitis virus and St Louis encephalitis virus.
- Rabies virus (migrates up peripheral nerves to the CNS, producing encephalomyelitis).

Neurological disorders

CLINICAL FEATURES

- **Symptoms**:
  - Inflammation of the brain parenchyma produces relatively non-specific symptoms such as irritability, altered personality, drowsiness and confusion.
  - Fever and headache occur early.
  - Rapid progression to focal neurological deficit may occur.
  - Seizures may occur.
  - Symptoms of meningism (see prior section) may occur due to concomitant inflammation of meninges (meningoencephalitis).
- **Signs**:
  - Focal neurology exists.
  - Brainstem involvement may produce cranial nerve palsies and a disrupted breathing pattern.
- **Rabies infection**:
  - Characterized by aching/pain at infection site.
  - Facial spasms are initiated by deep breaths or drinking (hydrophobia).
  - Myocarditis develops.
  - Ascending paralysis may occur.

INVESTIGATIONS

- **LP and CSF examination**:
  - Specific tests performed on CSF are as for meningitis; viral PCR is particularly important if encephalitis is suspected.
  - Red blood cells or xanthochromia may be present.
  - White cells will be elevated. HSV encephalitis will produce a similar profile to viral meningitis.
- **Imaging**: In HSV encephalitis, CT head may show lesions in temporal lobes, which enhance with contrast, although magnetic resonance imaging (MRI) is more sensitive.
- **Electroencephalogram**: may show abnormal activity arising from temporal lobes in HSV encephalitis.
- **Brain biopsy**: required for definitive diagnosis but normally not necessary in a case of HSV encephalitis with typical CT/MRI findings and a good response to treatment.

MANAGEMENT

Empirical antiviral agents should be started.
- **HSV**: Acyclovir IV 10 mg/kg every 8 hours for 21 days reduces mortality from 60–80% to less than 25%.
- **Arboviruses**: There is no specific treatment for encephalitis caused by an arbovirus. Clinical severity varies between arboviruses; Japanese B encephalitis has 20% mortality.

- **Rabies**: Once symptoms appear, death is inevitable. However, a protective vaccination is available, and post-exposure prophylaxis with wound cleaning and immunization is effective.

19.3 CEREBRAL ABSCESS

DEFINITION

- A cerebral abscess is a collection of pus within the cerebral hemispheres.

AETIOLOGY

- An abscess may result from spread of infection from a local site (e.g. sinusitis, otitis media, mastoiditis) or a distant site (e.g. endocarditis, discitis).
- An abscess may also complicate cranial trauma, including neurosurgery.
- Causative organisms include:
  - *Staphylococcus aureus*;
  - *Streptococcus pneumoniae*;
  - Viridans streptococci;
  - *Haemophilus influenza*;
  - *Pseudomonas aeruginosa*;
  - and mixed infection in up to 50% of cases.

CLINICAL FEATURES

- Symptoms and signs of intracranial mass including raised ICP, headache and altered consciousness.
- Seizures.
- Fever.
- Focal neurology related to the position of the abscess.

INVESTIGATIONS

- LP is **contraindicated** due to the risk of sudden decompression.
- Blood cultures.
- **Imaging**:
  - **CT head**: ring-enhancing lesions;
  - **MRI head**: achieves a better visualization of the posterior fossa.
- **Aspiration**: required to make a definitive diagnosis and identify the causative organism.

MANAGEMENT

- **Empirical treatment**:
  - cephalosporin: ceftriaxone, or if the abscess is a complication of a neurosurgical procedure, then ceftazidime is preferable;
  - metronidazole.

- Rationalise antibiotics when further microbiological evidence is available.
- Surgical drainage may be required.
- Corticosteroids may be used to reduce cerebral oedema.

19.4 DISCITIS AND EPIDURAL ABSCESS

- See Section 9.6.

19.5 HIV/AIDS AND OPPORTUNISTIC INFECTIONS

OVERVIEW

- HIV infection can produce a range of neurological complications.
- Mechanisms of neurological disease:
  1. Direct effect of HIV infection.
  2. Secondary infection with opportunistic organisms.
  3. Increased propensity to develop neoplasms.
- Similar opportunistic infections can also occur in other immunocompromised states.

DIRECT EFFECTS OF HIV INFECTION

- **Seroconversion illness**:
  - During the initial stage of HIV infection, a systemic 'flu-like' illness occurs.
  - Patients become asymptomatic when the immune system develops antibodies against the virus.
  - Seroconversion illness may include viral meningitis and a GBS-like acute inflammatory motor neuropathy.
- **HIV encephalopathy/AIDS dementia complex**:
  - These occur in 30–50% of patients with advanced AIDS.
  - HIV encephalopathy is suspected in early-onset dementia, with relatively symmetrical white matter hyperintensities on MRI.
- **Vacuolar myelopathy**: AIDS or advanced HIV can produce a myelopathy by damage to the white matter of the spinal cord; this may coincide with HIV encephalopathy.
- **Polyneuropathy**: HIV infection can produce a predominantly sensory peripheral neuropathy; however, this occurs more commonly as a side effect of antiretroviral medications.
- **Myopathy**:
  - Polymyositis can occur in HIV infection, possibly due to immune cross-reactivity.
  - In addition, zidovudine (AZT) can cause a proximal neuropathy.

OPPORTUNISTIC INFECTIONS IN AIDS

Cryptococcal meningitis
- See Section 19.1 discussion of fungal meningitis.

HSV/VZV encephalitis
- See Section 19.2.

Cytomegalovirus encephalitis
- This encephalitis is caused by cytomegalovirus.
- **Presentation**: Presents similarly to HIV encephalopathy but has a more rapid onset. Systemic CMV infection is often present. The III and VII cranial nerve palsies are particularly common.
- **Investigations**: CMV typically causes a ventriculitis that can be identified on MRI. The virus may be identified with PCR.
- **Management**: Intravenous ganciclovir and **highly active antiretroviral therapy** (HAART) should be given with the aim of restoring the CD4 count (see **Table 19.3**).

Cerebral toxoplasmosis
- Cerebral toxoplasmosis is caused by the protozoa *Toxoplasma gondii*.

CLINICAL FEATURES
- Subacute onset of fever and confusion is common; seizures and focal neurological deficit may also occur.

INVESTIGATIONS
- **CT head**: Ring-enhancing lesions are seen in cerebral and cerebellar hemispheres.
- **Serology**: Almost all patients are positive for *Toxoplasma* antigen.
- **Brain biopsy**: This is used for definitive diagnosis but may not be required.

MANAGEMENT
- High-dose pyrimethamine and sulphadiazine (or clindamycin) are given for 6 weeks, and then a maintenance dose will be required for life.

Table 19.3 **CD4 counts associated with neurological manifestations in HIV**

CD4 COUNT (CELLS/µL)	ASSOCIATED OPPORTUNISTIC INFECTION
<50	CMV encephalitis
<100	Cryptococcal meningitis, PML
<200	Cerebral toxoplasmosis, malignancy

Neurological disorders

- Antimicrobials are often used diagnostically as well as therapeutically with regular imaging to assess response.
- Corticosteriods may be used to reduce cerebral oedema.

Progressive multifocal leucoencephalopathy

- Progressive multifocal leucoencephalopathy (PML) is caused by reactivation of the JC virus.
- Typically, it presents with subacute or chronic visual and cognitive impairment.

DIAGNOSIS

- MRI is used; white matter lesions will be visible, particularly within the posterior region of the cerebral hemispheres.

MANAGEMENT

- Progression of the infection can be stopped by introducing HAART, but neurological deficit rarely improves.

HIV-RELATED MALIGNANCY

Primary CNS lymphoma

- A primary CNS lymphoma is the most common malignancy associated with HIV infection.
- Clinical presentation is typically with focal neurological deficit, confusion and headache.
- It can be difficult to distinguish from toxoplasmosis on imaging and should be considered if a case of suspected toxoplasmosis is not responding to a trial of antimicrobial medication.
- Brain biopsy will provide the definitive diagnosis. Prognosis is poor.

19.6 NEUROSYPHILIS

OVERVIEW/AETIOLOGY

- Syphilis is a sexually transmitted infection caused by the spirochete *Treponema pallidum*.
- Neurological disease is a feature of tertiary syphilis.
- It consists of three distinct syndromes:
  - **Meningovascular syphilis**:
    - This presents 2–5 years after the initial infection.
    - It can present as an acute meningitis but more commonly causes chronic basal meningitis associated with cranial nerve palsies.
    - Cerebral arteritis can lead to stroke.
  - **General paresis of the insane (GPI)**:
    - Meningoencephalitis and cerebral atrophy occur approximately 10 years after initial infection;

- – A severe deficit of higher cognitive function results, including confusion and seizures;
- – This is associated with a tremor of the mouth and tongue and hyperreflexia.
- **Tabes dorsalis**:
  - – This develops at least 20 years after the initial infection.
  - – Demyelination of the dorsal columns of the spinal cord produces sensory ataxia, altered vibration and soft touch sensation, prominent neuralgia and urinary incontinence.
  - – Cranial nerve palsies and autonomic neuropathy can also occur.
- Argyll Robertson pupil is caused by damage to the afferent fibres of the light reflex.

DIAGNOSIS

- Microscopy is performed of the primary chancre biopsy.
- Serology is required to diagnose secondary and tertiary infection.
- The venereal disease research laboratory (VDRL) and *Treponema pallidum* haemagglutination (TPHA) tests are older serology investigations that may be complementary to more modern serology.

INVESTIGATIONS (TABLE 19.4)

Table 19.4 Investigation findings in different stages of syphilis

STAGE OF DISEASE	VDRL	TPHA
Primary syphilis	+/-	+/-
Secondary syphilis	+	+
Tertiary syphilis	+/-	+
Treated syphilis	-	+

MANAGEMENT

- Neurosyphilis requires treatment with a 10-day course of intravenous penicillin.
- Treatment may produce some clinical improvement, but deterioration can still occur.

19.7 LYME DISEASE

DEFINITION/AETIOLOGY

- Lyme disease is a result of infection with the tick-borne spirochete *Borrelia burgdorferi*.
- It is associated with woodland areas that harbour ticks, particularly the New Forest in the United Kingdom.

Clinical features

- **Early localized infection** (1–30 days after bite): The first sign is often a characteristic spreading rash at the site of a tick bite (erythema chronicum migrans).
- **Early disseminated disease** (weeks to months after a bite):
  - **cardiovascular**: heart block;
  - **neurological** (neuroborrieliosis, 15% of cases): meningitis, a mild encephalitis and facial nerve palsy (most commonly);
  - **musculoskeletal**: migratory monoarthritis.
- **Chronic Lyme disease** (months to years after a bite):
  - **neurological**: subacute/chronic encephalomyelitis or a peripheral neuropathy;
  - **dermatological**: acrodermatitis chronica atrophicans, which is a rash over the extensor surfaces characterised by erythema and later atrophy.

Diagnosis

- **Microscopy**: Unlikely to identify the organism except very early in the disease course.
- **Serology**: Enzyme-linked immunosorbent assay (ELISA) allows detection of *Borrelia burgdorferi* antigens; it can take 4 weeks after infection to become positive.
- **CSF examination**: lymphocytic CSF in meningitis.
- **PCR**: on CSF, blood or synovial fluid.

Management

- If neurological disease is present, intravenous antibiotic therapy is required with ceftriaxone/cefotaxime or benzylpenicillin.
- In non-neurological disease, oral doxycycline or amoxicillin can be used.

19.8 CEREBRAL MALARIA

- Malaria is caused by infection with *Plasmodium* spp., protozoa transmitted by the bite of the female *Anopheles* mosquito.
- Cerebral involvement occurs rarely, usually in non-immune patients, and is almost exclusively caused by *Plasmodium falciparum*.

Clinical features

- Fever in a traveller returning from an endemic area should always prompt testing for malaria.
- Features specific to cerebral malaria include reduced level of consciousness, seizures and focal neurological deficit.

INVESTIGATIONS

- Thick and thin blood films identify the malarial parasite.
- Three negative films are required to exclude malaria.
- Antigen-detection methods are also available.

MANAGEMENT

- Cerebral involvement indicates severe malaria and requires treatment with intravenous quinine.
- A parasitaemia load greater than 10% or life-threatening organ failure, including coma, is an indication for plasma exchange (aiming to reduce the parasitaemia below 5%).
- Intensive care support may be required to manage renal failure, respiratory failure or coagulopathy.

19.9 POLIOMYELITIS

OVERVIEW/AETIOLOGY

- Poliomyelitis is an infection with one of the polioviruses, which usually cause diarrhoeal illness.
- Neurological disease results from infection of the anterior horn cells in the spinal cord or brainstem.
- Transmission is mainly faeco-oral, with some respiratory droplet spread.
- It has been eradicated in the developed world due to an effective vaccination program.

CLINICAL FEATURES

- In 0.1% of cases (more in adults), there is neurological involvement producing an asymmetrical flaccid paralysis with absent reflexes.
- Respiratory failure can develop.
- Sensation is unaffected.

DIAGNOSIS

- **PCR** detects poliovirus in respiratory secretions or stool.
- **CSF** examination reveals a lymphocytosis.

MANAGEMENT

- An effective vaccine is available for prevention.
- No specific treatment exists for neurological disease.
- Supportive measures may be required, especially respiratory support.
- Usually, a full recovery occurs, but patients may be left with long-standing neurological deficit.

Neurological disorders

19.10 MYCOBACTERIAL INFECTIONS

MYCOBACTERIUM TUBERCULOSIS

- Neurological disease includes:
    - tuberculous meningitis (see Section 19.1);
    - **tuberculomas**: mass lesions in the brain parenchyma or spinal cord that produce symptoms related to their local mass effect;
    - **vertebral osteomyelitis (Pott's disease)**: infection of the vertebrae that can cause secondary compression of the spinal cord.

MYCOBACTERIUM LEPRAE AND MYCOBACTERIUM LEPROMATOSIS

- Infection with either of *Mycobacterium leprae* or *Mycobacterium lepromatosis* can cause Hansen's disease (leprosy).
- Bacterial transmission is via the respiratory route.
- It is a common cause of polyneuropathy in the developing world.
- Two distinct clinical syndromes exist:
    - **Tuberculoid leprosy**:
        - This occurs in individuals who mount an effective immune response to mycobacterial infection.
        - The infection is confined to small areas of skin; hypopigmented patches occur, and damage to the afferent nerves supplying the area produces sensory loss.
    - **Lepromatous leprosy**:
        - An inadequate immune response results in widespread infection.
        - Large peripheral nerves are predominantly affected, producing sensorimotor polyneuropathy.

DIAGNOSIS

- Usually a clinical diagnosis is made.
- **Microscopy**: Acid-fast bacilli may be visible on skin scrapings in lepromatous leprosy.

MANAGEMENT

- Rifampicin and dapsone are the mainstays of treatment with clofazimine added in lepromatous leprosy.
- Six months of treatment is usually required.

19.11 PRION DISEASES

- Prions are infectious proteins with no genetic material.
- They cause neurodegenerative conditions known as spongiform encephalopathies because they transform brain tissue so it has a sponge-like histological appearance.

- Prions are unique in that they can be inherited, occur sporadically or be transmitted as infectious agents.

CREUTZFELD–JAKOB DISEASE

AETIOLOGY

- For Creutzfeld–Jakob disease (CJD), 85% of cases occur sporadically, 5% appear to show a familial inheritance, and the remaining cases suggest that the prion protein may be transmitted in bodily fluids (e.g. via neurosurgical instruments).
- **New variant CJD (vCJD)** is believed to be linked to bovine spongiform encephalopathy in cattle; the disease is thought to occur via ingestion of infected meat.

CLINICAL FEATURES

- Clinically, there is rapidly progressive dementia.
- Abnormalities of motor function occur, including pyramidal tract weakness, extrapyramidal signs and cerebellar dysfunction. Particularly notable is prominent myoclonus.
- There is visual loss.
- **vCJD** often occurs at an earlier age, typically young adulthood.

DIAGNOSIS

- Diagnosis is largely clinical.
- **MRI brain with diffusion weighted imaging (DWI)**: This is frequently abnormal, but other imaging may be unremarkable.
- **Electroencephalogram (EEG)**: This shows triphasic periodic complexes that are characteristic of sporadic CJD.
- **CSF**: The 14.3.3 protein and neuron-specific enolase (NSE) proteins are elevated.
- **Brain biopsy**: This is diagnostic if there is uncertainty, but equipment used for interventions will need specialized disposal due to the difficulty of killing the prion protein.

MANAGEMENT

- There is no specific treatment for CJD; management is currently supportive.

PROGNOSIS

- CJD is always fatal. The disease course is typically months in the sporadic form but may be over a year in vCJD.

Neurological disorders

MICRO-case

HSV encephalitis

A 23-year-old man was brought to the emergency department by ambulance after experiencing a seizure at home. This was witnessed by his girlfriend, who said that he initially became unresponsive and then started shaking his arms and legs. In the emergency department, he is very aggressive, which is abnormal for him, and he is disoriented in time and place. A collateral history taken from his girlfriend reveals that he has been complaining of a headache for the last 2 days and has been feeling feverish and has vomited several times. He is normally fit and well.

He had a temperature of 39.1°C and a pulse rate of 100. Other vital signs were unremarkable. Examination was difficult due to agitation, but he had normal power and reflexes throughout the upper and lower limbs, and sensation appeared to be intact. Cranial nerve examination was impossible due to the patient's condition, but pupils were equal and reactive to light.

He required sedation to undergo a CT scan, which showed no intracranial bleed or mass lesions, and the normal anatomy was not distorted. CSF analysis showed lymphocytosis (white cell count 350, 95% lymphocytes) and elevated protein of 1.1 g/l. The patient was started on intravenous acyclovir for presumed viral encephalitis. MRI performed later showed high signal in the temporal lobes, suggestive of HSV1 infection. This was later confirmed with positive PCR testing of the CSF. He makes a good recovery, and after completing 3 weeks of intravenous acyclovir treatment, does not have any residual neurological deficit.

Summary points

- Meningitis and encephalitis should always be considered in patients who present with headache, fever and signs of meningism, as well as less-specific features such as seizures and altered consciousness/aggression.
- Early administration of appropriate therapy reduces mortality and should not be delayed. Antibiotics and antiviral treatment should be started if the diagnosis is in doubt. Treatment can be rationalized based on the results of further investigations (e.g. CSF analysis, blood cultures).
- Brain imaging is required prior to LP in patients with altered consciousness, new focal neurology or signs of raised ICP.
- HSV1 is a treatable cause of encephalitis, so acyclovir should be used in all patients in whom encephalitis is suspected. The course of treatment may be reduced if HSV DNA is not isolated from the CSF.

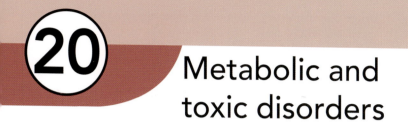

20 Metabolic and toxic disorders

20.1 OVERVIEW

- Systemic disturbance due to metabolic and toxic disorders often produces prominent neurological features.

20.2 METABOLIC DISTURBANCES DUE TO ORGAN FAILURE

CARDIOVASCULAR DISEASE

- Atrial fibrillation is the most common cause of embolic stroke (see Section 12.2).
- Temporary cardiovascular collapse and thus disruption of the blood supply to the brain will produce syncope and potentially permanent neurological deficit or seizures.

HEPATIC ENCEPHALOPATHY

- Hepatic encephalopathy is a symptom of decompensated liver failure; it results from high serum concentrations of ammonia (due to failure of the liver to metabolise nitrogenous waste).
- Decompensated liver failure commonly occurs in patients with chronic liver failure.
- Causes of acute decompensation include the following:
    - **increased gastrointestinal ammonia load**:
        - gastrointestinal bleeding;
        - constipation;
        - rarely a high-protein diet.
    - infection;
    - **increased concentration of blood ammonia**:
        - dehydration (including use of diuretics);
        - hypovolaemia.
    - renal failure;

- **drugs**: central nervous system (CNS) depressants may worsen hepatic encephalopathy:
  - opiates;
  - benzodiazepines;
  - anti-psychotics;
  - antidepressants.

CLINICAL FEATURES

Clinical features of hepatic encephalopathy

	CLINICAL FEATURES	ASTERIXIS?
Grade 0	Normal mental status, but there are subclinical changes in **concentration**, **memory, intellectual function** and **coordination**.	No
Grade 1	Grade 0 symptoms are more evident. In addition, patients may display **inappropriate moods and develop sleep disturbance**.	No
Grade 2	**Drowsiness**, gross cognitive deficit, disorientation in **time**.	Yes
Grade 3	**Drowsy but rousable, unable** to perform cognitive tasks, disorientation in **time and place**, **incomprehensible speech**.	Yes
Grade 4	Coma; may or may not respond to pain.	No

> ## MICRO-facts
>
> ### Asterixis
> Asterixis is a coarse, flapping tremor that can be seen in hepatic encephalopathy above **grade 2**; it disappears in **grade 4**.

DIAGNOSIS
- Diagnosis is mainly clinical.
- Serum ammonia will be elevated (>145 μmol/l).
- **Electroencephalogram (EEG)**: may show high-voltage triphasic slow waves.
- **Brain imaging**: important to rule out differential diagnoses.

MANAGEMENT
- Underlying precipitant should be identified and addressed.
- Avoid medications that can suppress CNS function.
- **Disaccharide lactulose**:
  - This stimulates tissues to pass ammonia into the gut lumen.

- Metabolism to lactic acid produces an acidic environment that inhibits ammonia-producing bacteria.
- Dosing should be titrated to produce two to four loose stools per day.
- **Antibiotics** (non-absorbable):
  - These reduce colonic concentrations of ammonia-producing bacteria.
  - Examples include metronidazole, neomycin or rifaximin.
- Low protein diet.
- **L-ornithine and L-aspartate (LOLA)**: increase the detoxification of ammonia into urea.
- **Intensive care**: Patients with grade 3 or 4 hepatic encephalopathy are at risk of aspiration and are likely to require intubation.

RENAL FAILURE

- Uraemia due to renal failure leads to the accumulation of neurotoxins.
- **Neurological clinical features**:
  - **Encephalopathy**:
    - insidious onset;
    - variable symptomology, including drowsiness, emotional disturbance and memory loss;
    - may display asterixis.
  - **Uraemic myopathy**: presents with proximal weakness.
  - **Polyneuropathy**: predominantly sensory peripheral neuropathy (see Section 10.4).

20.3 ENDOCRINE DISORDERS

THYROID DISEASE

- Both hypothyroidism and hyperthyroidism can produce a proximal myopathy and disturbance of cognition.
- **Hypothyroidism**:
  - slow relaxing reflexes and polyneuropathy;
  - liable to develop compression of the median nerve via a carpal tunnel syndrome.
- **Hyperthyroidism**: may produce a complex ophthalmoplegia via paralysis of the extraocular muscles.

DIABETES MELLITUS

- Diabetes is a strong risk factor for cerebrovascular disease (**see Section 12.1**); it is also a common cause of peripheral neuropathy (**see Section 10.4**).
- **Hyperosmolar hyperglycaemic state** (previously known as hyperosmotic non-ketotic—HONK)
  - This is associated with type II diabetes mellitus.

- Elevated serum glucose concentration causes an osmotic diuresis, and subsequent electrolyte disturbance may cause coma.
- **Hypoglycaemia**:
  - A common cause of altered consciousness;
  - Usually results from excessive dosing with anti-hyperglycaemic drugs.

20.4 ELECTROLYTE DISTURBANCES

- Hyponatraemia and hyper-/hypocalcaemia are important reversible causes of cognitive disturbance and seizures.
- Onset may be acute or even subacute with a dementia-like presentation.
- Severe or rapidly developing hyper- or hypokalaemia may produce muscle weakness.
- Inherited potassium channelopathies may cause intermittent weakness (periodic paralysis).

20.5 ALCOHOL-RELATED DISORDERS

ALCOHOL WITHDRAWAL

- Alcohol withdrawal is symptomatic in around half of all alcohol-dependent individuals after cessation of alcohol consumption.

CLINICAL FEATURES

- **Delirium tremens**:
  - **Autonomic symptoms**: These include sweating, palpitations and vomiting combined with agitation and hallucinations.
  - Hallucinations are classically visual and consist of small objects such as insects.
  - Approximately 2% of individuals will suffer seizures.

MANAGEMENT

- Reducing dose of a benzodiazepine such as chlordiazepoxide (lorazepam in hepatic impairment).
- Intravenous vitamin B complex (Pabrinex®) and oral thiamine to prevent Wernicke's encephalopathy.

WERNICKE'S ENCEPHALOPATHY AND KORSAKOFF'S SYNDROME

- Most common in alcoholics but may occur in patients who are malnourished for any reason (e.g. hyperemesis gravidarum).
- Caused by neuronal damage in the thalamus, brainstem, mamillary bodies and cerebellum due to deficiency of vitamin B_1 (thiamine).
- Often exacerbated by carbohydrate ingestion (carbohydrate metabolism requires thiamine).

CLINICAL FEATURES

- Presentation is classically a combination of one or more of the following:
  - ophthalmoplegia;
  - ataxia;
  - confusion (and impairment of short-term memory).

INVESTIGATIONS

- Usually, this is a clinical diagnosis; brain imaging is typically unremarkable.

MANAGEMENT

- Replacement of vitamin B_1, most often with intravenous Pabrinex® followed by oral thiamine.

COMPLICATIONS/PROGNOSIS

- Untreated mortality is approximately 20%.
- If the damage produced in Wernicke's encephalopathy becomes permanent, it develops into Korsakoff's syndrome:
  - Symptoms are similar but are not reversible with vitamin replacement.
  - Korsakoff's dementia results in severe anterograde amnesia with a degree of retrograde amnesia.
  - Patients typically confabulate (fill in gaps in memory with invented events); note that this is not a deliberate strategy.

20.6 PORPHYRIAS

- Porphyrias are a group of metabolic disorders caused by defects in the enzymes of the heme synthesis pathway.
- Usually, these are inherited but may rarely occur sporadically; the prevalence is estimated at 5 per 10,000.
- Symptoms arise because of the accumulation of toxic metabolites known as porphyrins and the deficiency of heme.
- Depending on the exact defect, the porphyrias have variable presenting features.
  - **Acute intermittent porphyria (AIP)**
    - AIP presents with acute episodes of abdominal pain associated with a mixed motor and sensory polyneuropathy and often psychiatric features. May also present as a seizure.
    - Acute attacks may be precipitated by medications, alcohol and infection.
  - **Porphyria cutanea tarda (PCT)**: presents chronically with a blistering rash on sun-exposed areas (often precipitated by acquired liver disease).

Neurological disorders

INVESTIGATIONS

- Urine:
  - Elevated porphyrins are present.
  - Patients with PCT will have red urine in natural light and purple urine in fluorescent light.
- Elevated porphyrin levels may also be detected in faeces and serum.
- Specific enzymatic assays and genetic testing will help to confirm the exact type of porphyria.

MANAGEMENT

- Acute porphyrias:
  - **intravenous glucose**: reduces the production of toxic porphyrins;
  - **intravenous heme**: replenishes deficiency and provides negative feedback on the disrupted synthesis pathway;
  - cessation of possible triggers;
  - treatment of underlying infection;
  - monitor for respiratory muscle weakness; some may require ventilatory support.
- Cutaneous symptoms:
  - avoidance of sunlight;
  - **venesection**: necessary in PCT due to accumulation of iron, which may result in haemochromatosis.

MICRO-case

Wernicke's encephalopathy

A 45-year-old man with a 2-day history of worsening confusion is brought to the emergency department by his brother. He smells strongly of alcohol, and vomits twice in the department. He has not had any falls, but his brother mentions that he seems to have been very unsteady on his feet over the past few days, although he usually can be a little unsteady when he is intoxicated. The patient denies any headache or fevers. A collateral history is taken from the brother, which reveals that the patient has been drinking up to 120 units of alcohol per week for the past 5 years. He tried to stop drinking a year prior but suffered significant withdrawal symptoms, including a seizure. His diet is very poor, with few regular meals.

On examination, the patient is disorientated in time and place, with a Glasgow Coma Scale (GCS) score of 14/15. He has marked nystagmus on ocular examination. There are no signs of meningism. Power and reflexes are normal throughout the limbs, although full neurological assessment is difficult due to poor patient compliance. Examination of the gait is not possible.

continued...

continued…

Investigations reveal moderately deranged liver enzymes but preserved liver synthetic function. Renal function and electrolytes are normal, but there is mild thrombocytopaenia and macrocytosis. A random blood glucose is 5.4 mmol/l. A chest radiograph and urinalysis are unremarkable. A computed tomographic (CT) scan of the brain shows no intracranial abnormality.

In light of the history of heavy alcohol intake, the patient is started on a reducing regime of oral chlordiazepoxide, and high-dose B complex vitamins (Pabrinex) are given intravenously. Over the next 2 days, the patient's confusion improves markedly, and his nystagmus resolves. A diagnosis of Wernicke's encephalopathy is made, and thiamine supplementation is continued. The patient is referred to the substance misuse team for further follow-up.

Summary points

- It is important to consider metabolic disturbances as a cause of acute or chronic neurological syndromes, including acute confusion and coma.
- Hypoglycaemia must be excluded in any patient with altered consciousness.
- Neurological disturbances are commonly seen in chronic alcohol excess, either due to acute withdrawal or deficiency states related to alcohol abuse.
- Vitamin B should be given to prevent or ameliorate neurological complications in **any** patient with a history of alcohol excess.

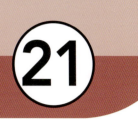

Neurological involvement in systemic disease and paraneoplastic syndromes

21

21.1 AUTOIMMUNE AND SYSTEMIC INFLAMMATORY DISORDERS

SYSTEMIC LUPUS ERYTHEMATOSUS

DEFINITION

- Systemic lupus erythematosus (SLE) is an autoimmune connective tissue disease with multisystem involvement.
- Neurological disease occurs in approximately 50%, and neurological complications are the third most common cause of death in SLE.

PATHOPHYSIOLOGY

- Affects the neurological system by a number of mechanisms:
  - **thrombophilia**: can affect arteries and veins, causing arterial stroke or venous sinus thrombosis;
  - **vasculitis**;
  - **encephalopathy**;
  - **myopathy**: secondary to vasculitis or due to primary myositis; also commonly caused by use of steroid medication in SLE;
  - **peripheral neuropathy**: secondary to vasculitis or directly from peripheral nerve demyelination.

NEUROLOGICAL CLINICAL FEATURES IN SLE

- Stroke (either arterial or venous in distribution).
- Seizures.
- Peripheral neuropathy (may involve the cranial nerves).
- Psychiatric symptoms, including depression, anxiety and frank psychosis.
- Myopathy with typical proximal weakness.

INVESTIGATIONS

- Diagnosis of SLE is according to clinical and laboratory features (diagnostic criteria available).
- **Blood tests**:
  - Results show raised inflammatory markers with anaemia/thrombocytopenia/leucopenia.

- **Autoantibodies**: Anti-dsDNA is specific for SLE. Other autoantibodies may also be present.
- **Neurological**:
  - **central nervous system (CNS) involvement**: magnetic resonance imaging (MRI) of the brain;
  - **peripheral nerves**: nerve conduction studies, electromyography (EMG) and muscle biopsy;
  - **cerebrospinal fluid (CSF)**: may show raised protein, white cells and oligoclonal bands.

Management

- The mainstay of therapy in SLE is immunosuppression.
- Corticosteroids may be useful acutely but are not appropriate in the long term due to side effects.
- Steroid-sparing agents are introduced as corticosteroids are weaned.
  - Hydroxychloroquine is a popular choice, particularly when SLE is limited to skin involvement.
  - Mycophenolate mofetil is better for widespread disease.
- Cyclophosphamide can be used acutely alongside corticosteroids.
- Monoclonal antibodies are being utilized with increasing frequency; the first choice in SLE is rituximab.
- If peripheral polyneuropathy is prominent, then therapy with intravenous immunoglobulin or plasma exchange is appropriate.
- Other neurological complications should be managed in a conventional fashion; seizures require anticonvulsant therapy, and thrombophilia will require anticoagulation.

SARCOIDOSIS

Definition

- Sarcoidosis is an inflammatory disorder of unknown cause characterised by the presence of non-caseating granulomas.
- This is a multisystem disorder, but it most commonly involves the lungs and intrathoracic lymph nodes; neurological involvement occurs in 5–10% of patients.

Clinical features

- Cranial nerve palsies are relatively common; sarcoidosis is the most common cause of bilateral lower motor neuron facial nerve palsies.
- Aseptic meningitis.
- Seizures.
- Peripheral neuropathy.
- Psychiatric symptoms.

INVESTIGATIONS

- Definitive diagnosis is made by tissue biopsy demonstrating non-caseating granulomas.
- **Chest X-ray**: may show bilateral hilar lymphadenopathy or interstitial lung disease.
- **Serum angiotensin converting enzyme (ACE) and calcium**: raised (representing granulomatous inflammation).
- **CSF analysis**: may show lymphocytosis, elevated protein and oligoclonal bands. CSF ACE level is of little diagnostic value.
- **MRI**: may show enhancing lesions consistent with an inflammatory process.

MANAGEMENT

- Corticosteroids are the mainstay of therapy for neurosarcoidosis.
- Other immunosuppressant therapies, including steroid-sparing agents such as methotrexate and biological agents such as infliximab (anti-TNF [tumour necrosis factor] antibody) have been reported to be effective in small numbers of patients.
- Symptomatic treatment of seizures and psychiatric manifestations is achieved using standard anticonvulsant and antipsychotic medication.

GIANT CELL ARTERITIS/TEMPORAL ARTERITIS

DEFINITION

- Giant cell arteritis (GCA)/temporal arteritis is a large-vessel vasculitis that predominantly affects the temporal arteries.
- Fifty per cent of patients also have polymyalgia rheumatica (PMR).

PATHOPHYSIOLOGY

- This is an autoimmune condition mediated via inflammatory cytokines.
- The underlying cause is unknown.
- The cytokine profiles involved in GCA and PMR are similar but not identical, suggesting that they represent associated but distinct disease processes.

EPIDEMIOLOGY

- Onset of GCA in individuals under the age of 50 is very rare.
- Estimated prevalence in individuals aged over 50 years is 20 per 100,000 in the United Kingdom. Increased prevalence occurs at more northern latitudes.
- It is more common in women than men (2:1).

NEUROLOGICAL CLINICAL FEATURES

- Involvement of branches of the external carotid artery:
    - causes unilateral headache, scalp tenderness and jaw claudication (pain on chewing or talking).

- Involvement of the ophthalmic artery (a branch of the internal carotid artery):
  - This may produce anterior ischaemic optic neuropathy (AION) with progressive visual loss due to disruption of the arterial supply to the optic nerve.
  - The extraocular muscles may also be affected, and visual loss may be preceded by diplopia.
  - Rarely, the arterial supply to the retina is affected, producing retinal ischaemia and typical changes on fundoscopy (pale retina with cherry red spot) with accompanying visual loss.
- Involvement of large arteries, including the aorta, is less common but can result in arm or leg claudication or even aneurysm formation.
- Half of patients with GCA also have symptoms of PMR, including pain and stiffness in proximal musculature. Classically, these symptoms are worse in the morning.

INVESTIGATIONS

- **Blood inflammatory markers**: Erythrocyte sedimentation rate (ESR) and C-reactive protein (CRP) are almost always raised. GCA may present without raised inflammatory markers, but this is uncommon.
- **Temporal artery biopsy** is the gold standard investigation but is only 80% sensitive due to skip lesions (areas of inflammation interspersed with normal tissue).
- Treatment is often started immediately, but temporal artery biopsy is still useful for 2 weeks; after that, detection of lesions is unlikely.

MANAGEMENT

- Oral steroids should be administered immediately on suspicion of giant cell arteritis and slowly weaned. The dose can be titrated to symptoms and blood inflammatory markers.
- Symptoms of GCA will resolve within a few weeks of steroid treatment; maintenance steroids are required for at least 2 years.
- Other immunosuppressive agents such as methotrexate and azathioprine may be used in resistant cases.
- Aspirin has been shown to reduce the risk of visual loss in GCA.

MICRO-print
Neurological vasculitis

- Neurological vasculitis affects the blood supply to nerves; it may be caused by GCA or any of the connective tissue disorders described or occur in isolation.

continued...

continued...

- In addition, any of the systemic vasculitides (e.g. Wegener's granulomatosis, polyarteritis nodosa, Churg-Strauss syndrome, Henoch-Scholein purpura, Beçhet's disease) may cause a CNS or peripheral nervous system (PNS) vasculitis.

Clinical features

- **Peripheral nerve vasculitis**: painful asymmetric motor sensory neuropathy, classically a **mononeuritis multiplex**.
- **CNS vasculitis**: focal neurological deficit, seizures, cognitive impairment and headache.
- Other symptoms, such as fever and weight loss, may also occur.
- Note that Beçhet's disease may produce a venulitis as well as an arteritis and can cause venous sinus thrombosis.

Investigations

- Inflammatory markers (except in isolated CNS vasculitis) are raised.
- Tissue biopsy where possible is the gold standard for diagnosis (peripheral nerve, meninges or muscle).
- Autoantibodies should be checked, but a negative anti-neutrophil cytoplasmic antibody (ANCA) does not rule out vasculitis.
- Four-vessel angiography (or magnetic resonance angiogram) is used to look for beading or strictures.

Management is with immunosuppression:

- Corticosteroids are commonly used in the acute phase (e.g. high-dose intravenous methylprednisolone).
- Other immunosuppressant agents include cyclophosphamide, mycophenolate and rituximab.

21.2 NEUROLOGICAL PARANEOPLASTIC SYNDROMES (TABLE 21.1)

- Paraneoplastic syndromes are disorders caused by a cancer but not by the direct physical effect of a tumour.
- They are mediated by antibodies, which are either produced by a tumour or produced by the immune system against the tumour but show cross-reactivity with host tissues.
- Early recognition can highlight the potential for underlying malignancy before it is clinically apparent and enable early detection and treatment.
- These syndromes are very rare, occurring in approximately 1% of cancers, but some tumours (e.g. small cell lung cancer) are particularly prone.

Neurological disorders

Table 21.1 Neurological paraneoplastic syndromes

SYNDROME	CLINICAL FEATURES	ASSOCIATED MALIGNANCIES	ASSOCIATED AUTOANTIBODIES
Limbic encephalitis	Severe progressive impairment of memory. Confusion, seizures and hallucination. Can be part of generalized encephalomyelitis.	Small-cell lung cancer (SCLC) Ovarian teratoma	**Anti-Hu** (SCLC) **Anti-NMDAR** (ovarian cancer)
Opsoclonus-myoclonus	Opsoclonus: random, chaotic movement of eyes. Can occur with myoclonus.	Children: neuroblastoma Adults: SCLC, breast cancer	**Anti-Ri** (breast carcinoma)
Cerebellar degeneration	Gait ataxia (progressing to truncal ataxia). Dysarthria, nystagmus and vertigo with vomiting can occur.	Gynaecological adenocarcinomas (ovary, uterus, etc.) Breast carcinoma SCLC Non-Hodgkin's lymphoma	**Anti-Yo** (gynaecological malignancies) **Anti-Hu** (SCLC) **Anti-Ri** (breast carcinoma)
Carcinoma-associated retinopathy	Loss of photore-ceptors causes intermittent visual problems, night blindness and colour vision impairment, progressing to visual loss.	SCLC	Anti-retinal antibodies
Sensory neuropathy	Pure sensory neuropathy. Painful sensory neuropathy. Mixed motor sensory neuropathy.	SCLC Breast carcinoma Prostate carcinoma	Anti-Hu
Lambert–Eaton syndrome	See Chapter 11, Neuromuscular junction and muscle.	Small-cell lung cancer	Anti-voltage-gated calcium channel

MICRO-case

Sarcoid neuropathy

A 47-year-old man presents to his general practitioner (GP) with a 2-day history of left-sided facial 'droop'. Six months previously, he was diagnosed with anterior uveitis. He also has an intermittent non-productive cough and occasional night sweats.

On examination, he has a left-sided lower motor neuron pattern facial weakness with normal sensation. There is purple swelling of the ears and nose, which the patient reports has been present for several years. There is no other focal neurology.

A chest X-ray shows bilateral hilar lymphadenopathy and serum calcium, and ACE levels are elevated.

A diagnosis of sarcoidosis is made, and the patient is commenced on high-dose corticosteroid treatment; his facial weakness recovers completely over the following weeks.

Summary point

- Systemic disease should be considered as a cause of neurological symptoms; autoimmune and inflammatory disorders can produce a wide range of neurological features and deficits.

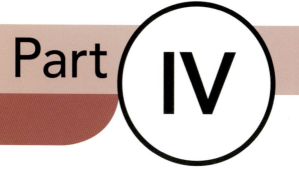

Part IV

Self-assessment:
Neurological zones

Self-assessment: Neurological disorders

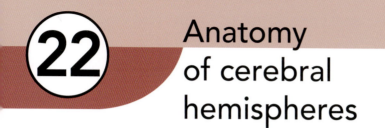

22 Anatomy of cerebral hemispheres

Questions

Diagnoses: EMQs

For each of the clinical scenarios that follow, choose the area within the brain most likely to be involved. Each answer may be used once, more than once or not at all.

Areas of the brain

1) Cerebellum
2) Left frontal lobe
3) Left parietal lobe
4) Left temporal lobe
5) Medulla
6) Pons
7) Right parietal lobe
8) Right occipital lobe
9) Right temporal lobe
10) Thalamus

Question 1

A 53-year-old plumber with a left homonymous hemianopia.

Question 2

A 53-year-old alcoholic with nystagmus and ataxia.

Question 3

An 82-year-old gentleman with expressive dysphasia.

Investigations: SBAs

For each of the following scenarios, select the intracranial structure most likely to be involved. Each answer may be used once, more than once or not at all.

Intracranial structures

1) Basilar artery
2) Left middle cerebral artery
3) Left middle meningeal artery
4) Left posterior cerebral artery

5) Left posterior communicating artery
6) Right cavernous sinus
7) Right middle cerebral artery
8) Right ophthalmic artery
9) Right posterior inferior cerebellar artery
10) Superior sagittal sinus

Question 4

A 34-year-old man with polycystic kidney disease and left oculomotor nerve palsy.

Question 5

A 23-year-old pregnant woman with headache, vomiting and ophthalmoplegia affecting the right eye.

Question 6

A 30-year-old rugby player who becomes drowsy and then unresponsive several hours after a blow to the head during a match. Computed tomography (CT) shows a left-sided biconvex haematoma with midline shift.

Answers

Diagnoses: EMQs

Answer 1

8) **Right occipital lobe**: A left homonymous hemianopia is a visual field defect affecting the entire left side of the visual field that results from damage to the right optic tract, in this case the right occipital lobe.

Answer 2

1) **Cerebellum**: Chronic alcohol abuse may lead to degeneration of the cerebellum, producing cerebellar signs such as ataxia, nystagmus and incoordination.

Answer 3

2) **Left frontal lobe**: Expressive dysphasia often represents a lesion affecting Broca's area, which is located in the dominant (usually left) frontal lobe.

Investigations: SBAs

Answer 4

5) **Left posterior communication artery**: An oculomotor nerve palsy may be the result of an aneurysm of the posterior communicating artery in the circle of Willis. Berry aneurysms are associated with polycystic kidney disease.

Answer 5

6) **Right cavernous sinus**: Headache and features of raised intracranial pressure in combination with cranial nerve palsies should raise suspicion of venous sinus thrombosis, especially in the context of a hypercoagulable state such as pregnancy. In this case, a cavernous sinus thrombosis is likely.

Answer 6

3) **Left middle meningeal artery**: A blow to the side of the head may tear the middle meningeal artery, causing arterial bleeding into the epidural space. This results in a haematoma contained by the skull sutures that appears biconvex on imaging. Patients classically have a lucid period following injury before developing reduced consciousness as the haematoma expands.

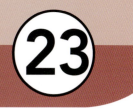

Basal ganglia and subcortical structures

23

Questions

Diagnoses: EMQs

Select the most likely cause for the following patients with abnormal movements. Each answer may be used once, more than once or not at all.

Options

1) Arteriosclerotic disease
2) Benign essential tremor
3) Hemiballismus
4) Huntington's disease
5) Idiopathic Parkinson's disease
6) Levodopa-induced dyskinesia
7) Multiple system atrophy
8) Progressive supranuclear palsy
9) Spasmodic torticollis
10) Wilson's disease

Question 7

A 21-year-old man is referred with a history of parkinsonian features and falls. On examination, he has parkinsonism, dysarthria and Kayser-Fleischer rings in his eyes. Initial investigations show abnormal liver function tests.

Question 8

A previously fit and well 67-year-old man presents with a 2-month history of slowly worsening shaking in his left hand, which disappears with movement. He also has difficulty walking, particularly downstairs. He is not on any medication. On examination, he has a resting tremor in his left hand with associated cogwheel rigidity in the left arm. He has a slow and shuffling gait and reduced right arm swing.

Question 9

A 54-year-old woman presents to her general practitioner (GP) with a 4-month progressive history of fatigue, unsteadiness and falls associated with dizziness on standing. On examination, she has parkinsonian features, severe postural hypotension and an ataxic gait.

Investigation: SBA

Question 10

A 65-year-old man presents with a tremor in his right hand and a history of frequent falls. On examination, he has parkinsonian features and dysarthria and is unable to follow the movement of objects in a vertical plane despite having normal ocular reflexes. He also appears slightly confused and scores 21 of 30 on a Mini-Mental State Examination (MMSE). What is the likely diagnosis? Please choose the single best answer from the following answers:

1) Alzheimer's dementia
2) Drug-induced parkinsonism
3) Huntington's disease
4) Idiopathic Parkinson's disease
5) Progressive supranuclear palsy

Answers

Diagnoses: EMQs

Answer 7

10) **Wilson's disease**: Wilson's disease is an autosomal recessive disorder affecting copper metabolism, and copper is deposited in the liver, basal ganglia, cornea and kidneys. A young patient presenting with liver disease or features of parkinsonism should be screened for Wilson's disease as it can be effectively treated.

Answer 8

5) **Idiopathic Parkinson's disease**: characterized by a classical triad of bradykinesia, rigidity and a resting tremor. Levodopa is effective for reducing bradykinesia and rigidity.

Answer 9

7) **Multiple system atrophy**: MSA is a progressive condition characterized by parkinsonian features, cerebellar ataxia and autonomic and urogenital dysfunction, including severe postural hypotension. It responds poorly to levodopa. Falls occur only late in the disease process in idiopathic Parkinson's disease, and cerebellar and autonomic features are not generally seen.

Investigation: SBA

Answer 10

5) **Progressive supranuclear palsy**: Parkinsonism combined with features not usually seen in idiopathic Parkinson's disease suggests one of the Parkinson's plus syndromes. The inability to track objects with the eyes suggests a gaze palsy, and this combined with the other features displayed by this gentleman points to progressive supranuclear palsy.

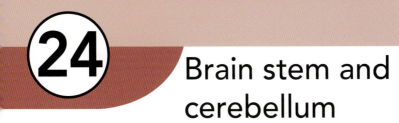

24 Brain stem and cerebellum

Questions

Diagnoses: EMQs

Based on the clinical scenarios, pick the most likely cranial nerve responsible for the patient's symptoms and signs. Each answer may be used once, more than once or not at all.

Cranial nerves

1) I Olfactory
2) II Optic
3) III Oculomotor
4) V Trigeminal
5) VI Abducens
6) VII Facial
7) VIII Vestibulocochlear
8) IX Glossopharyngeal
9) XI Spinal accessory
10) XII Hypoglossal

Question 11

A 21-year-old office worker presents to her GP with headaches and visual disturbance. The headaches started last week and are getting worse. She claims they are worse on standing and bending down and relieved by lying flat. She has an unremarkable past medical history, but her body mass index (BMI) is 36. Cranial nerve examination shows her inability to abduct her left eye. Retinal venous pulsation cannot be seen on fundoscopy.

Question 12

A 47-year-old gentleman presents to the emergency department with a suspected stroke. He feels well, apart from recovering from a recent viral illness. On examination, the right side of his face is droopy; he is unable to smile, blow out his cheeks or close his right eye. His facial sensation is normal. There are no other focal neurological signs on examination.

Question 13

A 77-year-old man with poorly controlled diabetes mellitus presents with severe double vision that was present on waking. On examination, his right eye is deviated down and out, and there is diplopia in all positions of gaze. The pupillary response is intact. The remainder of the examination reveals a reduced peripheral sensation but is otherwise normal.

Investigation: SBA

Question 14

A 45-year-old woman presents to her GP with a 4-week history of progressive unsteadiness when walking and difficulty with speech. On further questioning, she reveals significant weight loss and denies any dizziness or hearing loss. On examination, she has a marked intention tremor and past-pointing on the right side and displays nystagmus with the slow phase towards the left. A CT scan reveals a mass in the posterior fossa. Which of the following is the most likely site of the lesion? Please choose the single best answer from the following answers:

1) Cerebellopontine angle
2) Left cerebellar hemisphere
3) Medulla
4) Right cerebellar hemisphere
5) Superior vermis

Diagnoses: EMQs

Select the most likely diagnosis for each of the clinical scenarios that follow. Each answer may be used once, more than once or not at all.

Diagnostic options

1) Alcoholic cerebellar degeneration
2) Arnold–Chiari malformation
3) Cerebellar abscess
4) Cerebellar haemorrhage
5) Ethanol intoxication
6) Friedriech's ataxia
7) Hemangioblastoma
8) Multiple sclerosis
9) Paraneoplastic cerebellar degeneration
10) Wernicke's encephalopathy

Question 15

A 52-year-old man with a 20-year history of alcoholism presents to the emergency department with a 4-month history of progressive unsteadiness when walking. He is alert and oriented in time and place. He has impaired coordination on heel-shin testing bilaterally, but there is no intention tremor or past-pointing, and examination of the eyes is unremarkable. Tone and power in the limbs is normal. A CT scan shows cerebellar atrophy.

Question 16

A 13-year-old boy is brought to see his GP; he has a 1-year history of progressive problems with walking. He has been having problems with stumbling and tends to stand on widely spaced feet. His speech is jerky and spluttering. There is marked lower limb ataxia bilaterally with mild muscle weakness and wasting. Lower limb reflexes are absent, and sensory examination reveals absence of proprioception and vibration sense up to the level of the hips. Upper limb examination is normal. Moderate kyphoscoliosis is noted.

Question 17

A 62-year-old woman with a history of hypertension presents to the emergency department with a 1-hour history of sudden-onset severe headache with dizziness and neck stiffness. She is alert and oriented with a Glasgow Coma Scale (GCS) score of 15/15. Tone and power in all four limbs are normal, but she exhibits past-pointing and ataxia on the right side. Over the next few hours, her GCS drops to 13/15, and her plantars become extensor.

Answers

Diagnoses: EMQs

Answer 11

5) **VI abducens nerve**: This history points towards the diagnosis of benign intracranial hypertension. The patient's inability to abduct her left eye is due to compression of the abducens nerve due to raised intracranial pressure and is a false localizing sign. This patient will require a CT head scan to rule out other pathology and a lumbar puncture to reduce the pressure to try to preserve the patient's sight.

Answer 12

6) **VII facial nerve**: This history is relatively common and most likely represents a facial nerve palsy/Bell's palsy. The most common cause is herpes zoster. This patient does not require complex brain imaging but should be given advice regarding eye care and prescribed a week of steroids.

Answer 13

3) **III oculomotor nerve**: The examination findings in this gentleman point to a right oculomotor nerve palsy. Given his age, history of diabetes and absence of other neurological deficit, the most likely cause is microvascular infarction (may spare parasympathetic fibres and so pupillary response is unaffected).

Investigation: SBA

Answer 14

4) **Right cerebellar hemisphere**: These features are suggestive of a lesion of the right cerebellar hemisphere as cerebellar lesions produce ipsilateral signs. Lesions of the midline vermis produce gait and truncal ataxia, and cerebellopontine lesions may compress the cerebellum and produce signs, but usually cause hearing loss and dizziness as prominent features. Given the presence of a mass on imaging, this is likely to be due to metastases.

Diagnoses: EMQs

Answer 15

1) **Alcoholic cerebellar degeneration**: The absence of nystagmus and confusion as well as the slowly progressive course suggests a diagnosis of alcoholic cerebellar degeneration in this case rather than Wernicke's encephalopathy.

Answer 16

6) **Friedreich's ataxia**: Progressive gait ataxia presenting in early life is suggestive of an inherited ataxia. The combination of cerebellar ataxia (including gait and lower limb ataxia) and dysarthria with motor and sensory deficits suggests a diagnosis of Friedreich's ataxia. The presence of a skeletal abnormality is consistent with this.

Answer 17

4) **Cerebellar haemorrhage**: Sudden onset of headache with vestibular symptoms is suggestive of a vascular event affecting the cerebellum. Haemorrhage into one of the cerebellar hemispheres produces ipsilateral limb ataxia, and consciousness may become depressed as a bleed extends. Over time, haemorrhage also produces a mass effect, and compression of the brainstem explains the development of extensor plantars and reduced consciousness.

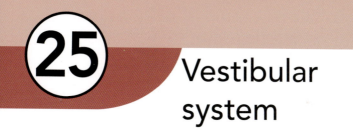

Vestibular system

Questions

Diagnoses: EMQs

Select the most likely diagnosis for each of the clinical scenarios that follow. Each answer may be used once, more than once or not at all.

Diagnostic options

1) Benign paroxysmal positional vertigo
2) Cerebellar abscess
3) Cerebellar stroke
4) Cerebellar tumour
5) Lateral medullary syndrome
6) Left acoustic neuroma
7) Ménière's disease
8) Meningioma
9) Right acoustic neuroma
10) Vestibular neuronitis

Question 18

A 48-year-old teacher presents to her GP having developed vertigo over the past week. She has noticed a progressive decline in her hearing over the past year. She is normally fit and well. On examination, you observe multiple small painless nodules all over her body and five café-au-lait spots. She has a sensorineural hearing loss on the left side and a fine tremor on the left with associated ataxia.

Question 19

A 58-year-old secretary requests a home visit from the GP as she feels too unwell to get to the surgery. On visiting, she is lying very still in bed. She describes a 2-day history of severe vertigo and nausea every time she moves her head. On the limited examination she allows you to do, you find nystagmus, and she remains dizzy throughout.

Question 20

A 32-year-old woman presents to her GP complaining of deafness. She is struggling to hear her clients, and some of her workmates have commented on her hearing loss. She describes dullness to her hearing, with a feeling of fullness within her ear. She also has some associated vertigo and an "annoying whooshing sound" in her ear. She also complains of feeling sick regularly. Her mother suffered from a condition that rendered her nearly deaf.

Answers

Diagnoses: EMQs

Answer 18

6) Left acoustic neuroma: This history is consistent with acoustic neuroma, which given the additional examination findings, is likely a result of neurofibromatosis. This patient will require imaging to determine the size of the tumour and the potential for resection.

Answer 19

10) Vestibular neuronitis: This is most likely acute vestibular neuronitis. It is an acute onset with persistent vertigo, and she feels unwell; therefore, benign paroxysmal positional vertigo (BPPV) is unlikely. The fact that she reports no hearing loss would make Ménière's disease and acoustic neuroma unlikely.

Answer 20

7) Ménière's disease: The family history is a subtle clue, but the triad of hearing loss, tinnitus and vertigo should make you suspect Ménière's disease. This patient will however require brain imaging to rule out acoustic neuroma. She should be treated with vestibular sedatives and supportive therapy, with a view to surgery if her symptoms continue to deteriorate. There is no cure for Ménière's disease.

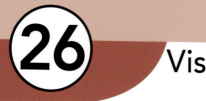

26 Visual tracts

Questions

Investigations: SBAs

Question 21

A 58-year-old man is seen in the neurology clinic following referral by his GP for a slowly progressive visual field defect. This has been accompanied by the onset of partial seizures and headaches. Magnetic resonance imaging (MRI) of his brain has shown a mass in the right temporal lobe, suggestive of a glioma. Which visual defect is this patient most likely to be experiencing? Please choose the single best answer from the following answers:

1) Bitemporal hemianopia
2) Congruent right homonymous hemianopia
3) Left central scotoma
4) Left homonymous lower quadrantanopia
5) Left homonymous upper quadrantanopia

Question 22

A 67-year-old woman presents to her GP with a 6-hour history of painless visual loss affecting her left eye. She has had increasingly severe left-sided headaches for the past 3 weeks, and her scalp is very tender to touch. She also notes that her jaw cramps up when she chews her food. On examination, she has a tender palpable left temporal artery, and the left optic disc appears slightly swollen. What is the most likely diagnosis? Please choose the single best answer from the following answers:

1) Amaurosis fugax
2) Anterior ischaemic optic neuropathy
3) Leber's optic neuropathy
4) Optic neuritis
5) Pituitary apoplexy

Question 23

A 61-year-old man attends his GP with a 2-month history of worsening problems with bumping into objects around the house. He notes that he tends to bump into things on his right-hand side. On examination, he has an incongruent right homonymous hemianopia, which is confirmed with formal visual field testing. Which of the following is the most likely site of the lesion that is causing this patient's visual field defect? Please choose the single best answer from the following answers:

1) Left occipital cortex
2) Left optic tract
3) Optic chiasm
4) Right optic nerve
5) Right optic tract

Question 24

A 27-year-old woman presents to her GP with a 2-day history of visual loss and pain affecting her right eye, which came on over the course of a day. She says that she noticed that colours became less prominent before her vision deteriorated. She reports that she had a similar episode a year previously, and that she has experienced an episode of transient weakness affecting her legs during the past 6 months. Which of the following is the most likely diagnosis? Please choose the single best answer from the following answers:

1) Anterior ischaemic optic neuropathy
2) Benign intracranial hypertension
3) Optic neuritis
4) Pituitary adenoma
5) Toxic optic neuropathy

Answers

Investigations: SBAs

Answer 21

5) **Left homonymous upper quadrantanopia**: Fibres of the optic radiation representing the lower half of the retina pass through the temporal lobe (known as Meyer's loop). A mass compressing these fibres in the right temporal lobe will produce a left homonymous upper quadrantanopia.

Answer 22

2) **Anterior ischaemic optic neuropathy**: This lady's history of sudden painless visual loss combined with a story suggestive of temporal artery

inflammation points to the diagnosis of anterior ischaemic optic neuropathy due to giant cell arteritis. As the visual loss has not resolved rapidly, amaurosis fugax is excluded, and optic neuritis is classically painful and has a slower onset. Pituitary apoplexy would produce a bitemporal hemianopia rather than unilateral visual loss.

Answer 23

2) **Left optic tract**: A right homonymous hemianopia is caused by a left-sided visual tract lesion. The fact that the defect is incongruous points to a lesion of the left optic tract of the lateral geniculate nucleus. A lesion of the right optic nerve would produce unilateral visual loss, and a lesion of the occipital cortex would cause a highly congruent homonymous hemianopia.

Answer 24

3) **Optic neuritis**: This history is highly suggestive of optic neuritis. This lady appears to have had a previous episode of optic neuritis and what sounds like transient paraparesis; these relapsing and remitting neurological episodes may suggest an underlying diagnosis of multiple sclerosis. Idiopathic intracranial hypertension (IIH) and a pituitary adenoma are likely to cause a bilateral visual field defect. The speed of onset of the visual disturbance excludes vascular and degenerative causes.

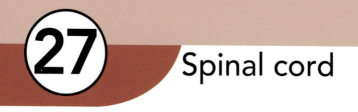

Questions

Diagnoses: EMQs

From the investigations listed, choose the single most appropriate one for each clinical scenario to determine the diagnosis. Each answer may be used once, more than once or not at all.

Investigations

1) Autoantibody screen
2) CT head
3) CT spine
4) Erythrocyte sedimentation rate (ESR) and C-reactive protein (CRP)
5) Haematinics
6) MRI spine
7) Nerve conduction studies and electromyogram
8) Positron emission tomographic (PET) scan
9) Plain spine X-rays
10) Transcranial magnetic stimulation

Question 25

A 49-year-old builder is referred by his GP for worsening back pain. He has had lumbar back pain for the past 3 months, but on waking this morning, the pain was much more intense, stabbing in nature with no radiation. He has tried simple analgesia with no relief. He also complains of being unable to pass urine, despite feeling that he needs to do so. On examination, he also has saddle anaesthesia.

Question 26

A 56-year-old woman is referred to a neurologist by her GP. She has developed progressive weakness of her right leg over the past 12 months, and her walking is now impaired. On examination, there is muscle wasting, fasciculation and weakness in the right leg and to a lesser degree in the left leg and the right arm. Reflexes are brisk in all four limbs. Sensation is unaffected.

Question 27

A 76-year-old gentleman is admitted to the hospital with severe back pain, ongoing for the past week, and feeling generally unwell. His past medical history reveals that he has a pacemaker inserted for heart block, and he is known to have mild mitral stenosis. On examination, he has a low-grade fever of 37.4°C, a loud ejection systolic murmur, and severe tenderness on palpation over the T12 and L1 vertebrae. He has no weakness of his arms or legs; tone and reflexes are normal, but he has severe pain on trying to sit up. His CRP is 312, and an echocardiogram shows mitral valve vegetation. Blood cultures subsequently grow a *Streptococcus* species. Plain films are taken of the spine, but there are no obvious abnormalities.

Answers

Diagnoses: EMQs

Answer 25

6) **MRI spine**: the appropriate investigation is an urgent MRI spine; these are the symptoms of the cauda equina syndrome; without timely intervention, urological function may be permanently impaired. A neurosurgical opinion regarding decompression as a matter of urgency is required if cauda equina syndrome is confirmed to give the patient the best chance of recovery.

Answer 26

7) **Nerve conduction studies and electromyogram**: A combination of upper and lower motor neuron signs and the absence of any sensory symptoms are highly suggestive of motor neuron disease affecting the ventral horn. The most appropriate investigation is nerve conduction studies and electromyogram, but MRI spine will be important to rule out differential diagnoses.

Answer 27

8) **PET scan**: This presentation suggests discitis, likely resulting from infectious emboli from an endocardial vegetation. An MRI spine should be performed; however, due to the pacemaker, this is not possible. Therefore, a PET scan is indicated. This patient will require bed rest for 2 weeks to prevent kyphotic deformity and a spinal brace for up to 6 weeks, as well as long-term antibiotic therapy.

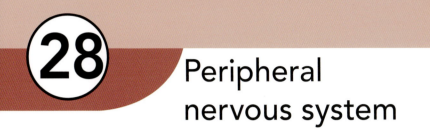

Peripheral nervous system

Questions

Diagnoses: EMQs

Select the most likely diagnosis for each of the clinical scenarios that follow. Each answer may be used once, more than once or not at all.

Diagnostic options

1) Carpal tunnel syndrome
2) Complex partial seizure
3) Diabetic amyotrophy
4) Diabetic neuropathy
5) Drug-induced neuropathy
6) Guillain–Barré syndrome
7) Ulnar nerve entrapment
8) Uraemic neuropathy
9) Vasculitic mononeuritis multiplex
10) Vitamin B_{12} deficiency

Question 28

A 37-year-old man with a long history of changeable bowel habit and abdominal pain presents with a 5-month history of worsening tingling and burning pain in his hands and feet. On examination, he has no weakness or wasting of the distal limb muscles, and Romberg's sign is negative, although he has impairment of vibration sense and proprioception in a glove-and-stocking distribution. Investigations reveal a macrocytic anaemia (mean corpuscular volume [MCV] 102).

Question 29

A 64-year-old man with recent diagnosis of type 2 diabetes sees his GP; the man complains of severe pain in his thighs that has been troubling him for the last 4 weeks. He has also found that walking has become more difficult; especially, he struggles with going up stairs and finds his feet often catch on the steps. On examination, he has demonstrable weakness of his quadriceps muscles and hip flexors, which are also wasted. The knee reflexes are absent. He has a very mild sensory impairment affecting the soles of his feet. His HbA1c is 9%.

Question 30

A 41-year-old bricklayer presents to his GP with a 2-month history of numbness and problems with gripping in his left hand. He complains that he cannot fully extend his little and ring fingers, and this is interfering with his work. On examination, he has wasting of the medial forearm muscles and hypothenar eminence and moderate clawing of the medial two fingers of his left hand. There is reduced sensation over the medial aspect of the palm, and his grip strength is reduced. He does not have any other neurological deficit.

Investigations: SBAs

Question 31

A 46-year-old woman complains of a 3-month history of shooting pains and tingling affecting the thumb, first two fingers and the lateral aspect of the palm of her right hand. Her symptoms are worse at night. Her GP suspects carpal tunnel syndrome is the likely diagnosis. Which of the following is *not* associated with carpal tunnel syndrome? Please choose the single best answer from the following answers:

1) Alcohol abuse
2) Hypothyroidism
3) Obesity
4) Pregnancy
5) Rheumatoid arthritis

Question 32

A 26-year-old man is brought to the emergency department with rapidly ascending weakness affecting his upper and lower limbs. Three weeks ago, he had a viral illness that was diagnosed as infectious mononucleosis, and in the past week, he has been experiencing pain between his shoulders. He is admitted to the neurology unit with suspected Guillain–Barré syndrome. Which of the following is true concerning Guillain–Barré syndrome? Please choose the single best answer from the following answers:

1) It is a rare cause of non-traumatic paralysis.
2) It is highly responsive to corticosteroid treatment.
3) The peak of severity of clinical features occurs within 4 weeks of onset.
4) There is an association with *Streptococcus pneumoniae* infection.
5) There is equal motor and sensory deficit.

Question 33

A 27-year-old man with several previous psychiatric admissions is admitted under the surgeons' care with abdominal pain. On further examination, he has mixed peripheral neuropathy with no other abnormalities, and a neurology opinion is requested. Initial investigations, including a blood film, are normal. Further specialized tests confirm the diagnosis. What is the most likely diagnosis? Please choose the single best answer from the following answers:

1) Acute intermittent porphyria
2) Diabetic neuropathy
3) Guillain–Barré syndrome
4) Hereditary motor-sensory neuropathy
5) Lead poisoning

Answers

Diagnoses: EMQs

Answer 28

10) Vitamin B$_{12}$ deficiency: This history is highly suggestive of polyneuropathy. Vibration sense and proprioception are usually the first sensory modalities to be affected in small-fibre neuropathy. **Vitamin B$_{12}$ deficiency** is a common cause of peripheral neuropathy and macrocytic anaemia. Causes of vitamin B$_{12}$ deficiency are various but include Crohn's disease, which may the case here.

Answer 29

3) Diabetic amyotrophy: The severe pain in the thighs accompanied by weakness and wasting of the knee extensors and hip flexors suggests diabetic amyotrophy. His poor glycaemic control is demonstrated by his high HbA1c value of 9%, which equates to an average glucose concentration of around 12 mmol/l.

Answer 30

7) Ulnar nerve entrapment: The involvement of the forearm muscles suggests ulnar nerve entrapment at the elbow. Recovery may occur with rest and splinting of the elbow in extension; alternatively, surgical decompression of the cubital tunnel may be required. Clawing of the medial two fingers occurs due to the paralysis of the interossei and medial two lumbrical muscles, which allows hyperextension of the MCP joints. The severity of clawing increases with more distal ulnar nerve injury.

Investigations: SBAs

Answer 31

1) Alcohol abuse: All of the options apart from alcohol abuse are associated with carpal tunnel syndrome. Alcohol abuse is associated with other forms of neuropathy.

Answer 32

3) **Guillain–Barré syndrome**: The peak severity of clinical features occurs within 4 weeks of onset.

Guillain–Barré is the most common non-traumatic cause of paralysis in the Western world and is particularly associated with *Campylobacter jejuni* gastroenteritis. It not responsive to corticosteroid treatment, and it usually produces a motor-predominant deficit. The most dangerous symptom of Guillain–Barré is respiratory failure; it is essential to closely monitor the forced vital capacity (FVC) and provide ventilatory support if required.

Answer 33

1) **Acute intermittent porphyria**: This is the most likely diagnosis and could be confirmed by checking blood and urine porphyrins. The history is not typical for diabetic neuropathy or hereditary motor-sensory neuropathy. Guillain–Barré is a possibility; however, Guillain–Barré does not reoccur, and it would not explain the psychiatric symptoms. Lead poisoning would produce a microcytic anaemia and basophilic stippling of red blood cells on the blood film.

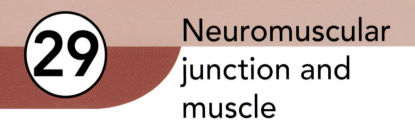

29 Neuromuscular junction and muscle

Questions

Investigations: EMQs

Question 34

A 52-year-old woman is seen by her GP after complaining of worsening weakness of her legs; she says she now has difficulty walking, and that her legs feel very heavy. She finds that her symptoms improve after she has used her rowing machine. She also complains of a dry mouth for the last few weeks. She is a heavy smoker and has lost several kilograms in weight over the last 2 months. On examination, she has very mild ptosis and no diplopia. Which of the following is the single most likely diagnosis? Please choose the single best answer from the following answers:

1) Guillain–Barré syndrome
2) Lambert–Eaton myaesthenic syndrome
3) Motor neuron disease
4) Myaesthenia gravis
5) Syringomyelia

Question 35

A 46-year-old man is admitted to the neurology unit with rapidly worsening fatigable weakness and recent onset of difficulty breathing. It is thought he is having a myaesthenic crisis, and diagnosis of myasthenia gravis is made. Which of the following is a feature of myasthenia gravis? Please choose the single best answer from the following answers:

1) Marked sensory disturbance
2) No response to administration of edrophonium
3) Presence of a thymoma
4) Presence of antibodies to voltage-gated calcium channels.
5) Weakness worse first thing in the morning

Question 36

Which of the following clinical features is *not* seen in myasthenia gravis?
Please choose the single best answer from the following alternatives:

1) Diplopia
2) Dry mouth
3) Dysphagia
4) Muscle wasting
5) Ptosis

Diagnoses: EMQs

**Select the most likely diagnosis for each of the clinical scenarios that
follow. Each answer may be used once, more than once or not at all.**

Diagnostic options

1) Acid maltase deficiency
2) Dermatomyositis
3) Drug-induced myopathy
4) Duchenne muscular dystrophy
5) Guillain-Barré syndrome
6) Hypokalaemic periodic paralysis
7) Hypothyroidism
8) Limb girdle dystrophy
9) Myotonic dystrophy
10) Polymyositis

Question 37

A 27-year-old woman presents to her local walk-in centre with a 3-week
history of pain and weakness in the muscles of her thighs and upper arms.
She describes difficulty washing her hair and picking up her young child.
She has also noticed a rash over her chest and arms. On examination, she has
weakness and wasting of the pelvic and shoulder girdle muscles and marked
muscle tenderness. The distal muscles are normal. She appears to have a purple
discoloration around her eyes. Blood tests reveal an ESR of 37 mm/hour and a
CPK of 1250 U/l.

Question 38

A 51-year-old man presents to his GP with severe pain in his thighs that has
come on over the last 3 days. He has noticed problems with climbing the stairs
at home but does not think his legs are especially weak. On examination,
there is tenderness of the quadriceps muscles and reduced power of hip flexion
and knee extension, although some of this is due to pain. There is no distal
weakness, and sensation is intact. The GP notices that one of his partners
started the patient on a tablet for high cholesterol 2 weeks ago.

Question 39

A 22-year-old man presents to his GP after noticing that when he shakes
hands with people he finds it difficult to let go. On questioning, he says

that his grip strength has reduced over the past year. His girlfriend, who accompanies him, also says that his facial appearance has changed somewhat over the past 18 months, and his face now looks 'thinner' than previously. She thinks he sleeps a lot during the day despite sleeping well at night. Examination reveals muscle weakness and wasting of distal and facial muscles.

Investigations: SBAs

Question 40

A 38-year-old woman is admitted to the neurology unit for investigation of muscle tenderness and proximal weakness. Which of the following features is *not* consistent with a diagnosis of polymyositis? Please choose the single best answer from the following answers:
1) Anti-Jo1 antibodies
2) Necrosis of muscle fibres on biopsy
3) No response to corticosteroids or other immunosuppression
4) Normal ESR
5) Raised serum creatine kinase

Question 41

A 5-year-old boy with walking problems is seen in clinic. He had previously been able to run, but over the last year has become unable to do so. His parents have also noticed that he has trouble standing up from the floor after playing with toys and has to walk his hands up his body. The neurologist suspects a diagnosis of Duchenne muscular dystrophy. Which of the following is not a feature of Duchenne muscular dystrophy? Please choose the single best answer from the following answers:
1) X-linked recessive inheritance
2) Calf pseudohypertrophy
3) Elevated serum creatine kinase
4) Ocular muscle involvement
5) Presents in early childhood

Answers

Investigations: EMQs

Answer 34

2) **Lambert–Eaton myaesthenic syndrome**: The history is typical of the Lambert–Eaton myaesthenic syndrome. This produces a proximal weakness

that improves briefly with exertion. Ocular muscles are relatively spared compared to myasthenia gravis, and autonomic involvement can occur. Lambert–Eaton is usually a paraneoplastic syndrome caused by anti-voltage-gated calcium channel antibodies produced by small-cell lung cancer.

Answer 35

3) Presence of a thymoma: A thymoma or thymus hyperplasia occurs in up to 75% of cases of myasthenia gravis; removal of a thymoma can be curative. Antibodies against voltage-gated calcium channels are a feature of Lambert–Eaton; sensory disturbance is not a feature of myasthenia gravis, and weakness tends to deteriorate towards the end of the day with activity. Edrophonium is used in the tensilon test; this anticholinesterase agent typically produces a rapid transient improvement in weakness.

Answer 36

2) Dry mouth: All of the listed features are seen in myasthenia gravis with the exception of dry mouth, which is an autonomic symptom that is seen in Lambert–Eaton myaesthenic syndrome.

Diagnoses: EMQs

Answer 37

2) Dermatomyositis: This presentation is suggestive of inflammatory myopathy. The purple discolouration around the eyes is likely to be the heliotrope rash seen in dermatomyositis. The markedly raised CPK supports this diagnosis.

Answer 38

3) Drug-induced myopathy: This patient has features of an inflammatory myopathy, and the recent introduction of a new drug should prompt suspicion of a drug-induced myopathy. Statins are one of the most common causes of drug-induced myopathies; stopping the drug should resolve the symptoms.

Answer 39

9) Myotonic dystrophy: This patient has features of chronic myopathy. Myotonic dystrophy causes wasting and weakness of the distal limb and facial muscles, which produces a typical myotonic appearance. Intellectual slowing and hypersomnolence are also features. Age of onset varies according to the expanded allele size, with most affected individuals showing signs in early adulthood.

Investigations: SBAs

Answer 40

3) **No response to corticosteroids or other immunosuppression**: All of the features listed are found in polymyositis with the exception of a poor response to immunosuppression. Anti-Jo1 antibodies are seen in a minority of cases of polymyositis and are a predictor of poor prognosis. The ESR is usually raised in inflammatory myopathies, but a normal value does not exclude the diagnosis.

Answer 41

4) **Ocular muscle involvement**: Duchenne muscular dystrophy always presents in early childhood, and inheritance is X-linked. There is massive elevation of serum creatine kinase, and calf pseudohypertrophy occurs due to fatty infiltration of muscle. Ocular muscle involvement does not occur in Duchenne muscular dystrophy.

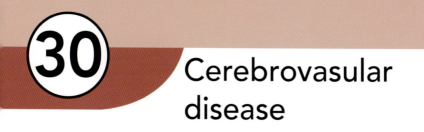

30 Cerebrovasular disease

Questions

Diagnoses: EMQs

Select the most likely diagnosis for the following patients with stroke. Each answer may be used once, more than once or not at all.

Diagnostic options

1) Anterior cerebral artery territory infarction
2) Basilar artery dissection
3) Cerebellar haemorrhage
4) Lacunar infarct of the internal capsule
5) Lateral medullary syndrome
6) Locked-in syndrome
7) Middle cerebral artery territory infarction
8) Pontine haemorrhage
9) Transient ischemic attack
10) Weber's syndrome

Question 42

A 65-year-old man with type 2 diabetes presents to the emergency department with sudden onset of vertigo, vomiting, double vision and hiccups. He is also having problems swallowing, and the right side of his face 'feels different'. On examination, he has impaired pain and temperature sensation over the right side of his face and right-sided Horner's syndrome. He has loss of pain and temperature sensation in the left side of his body and mild ataxia of the right limb. Over the next month, he makes a full recovery.

Question 43

A 58-year-old male with a long-standing history of hypertension presents in the emergency department with sudden collapse. He is unconscious and has a Glasgow Coma Scale (GCS) score of 4. On examination, he has pinpoint pupils, decerebrate posturing and bradypnoea.

Question 44

A 77-year-old hypertensive female develops an acute onset of severe weakness in her left side involving her lower face, arm and leg. On examination, she has left hemiplegia with no sensory loss. She has a GCS score of 15.

For each of the following clinical scenarios, please choose the blood vessel most likely to be involved. Each answer may be used once, more than once or not at all.

Options

1) Left anterior cerebral artery
2) Left internal carotid artery
3) Left middle cerebral artery
4) Left posterior cerebral artery
5) Left posterior inferior cerebellar artery

6) Right anterior cerebral artery
7) Right internal carotid artery
8) Right middle cerebral artery
9) Right posterior cerebral artery
10) Right posterior communicating artery

Question 45

A 68-year-old female with a long history of cardiovascular disease and high cholesterol suddenly becomes unsteady on her feet whilst doing her gardening. On examination in the emergency department, it is noted that she has some cuts and bruises on her right knee, but the left appears relatively unscathed. Power is reduced in the right leg but normal in the left leg and upper limbs.

Question 46

A 74-year-old right-handed male presents to the emergency department after his wife becomes concerned that he is unable to smile normally, does not understand what she is saying to him, and is unable to use his right arm. On examination, the patient has a right-hand-side facial droop and reduced power in his right arm and leg.

Question 47

A 74-year-old male goes to see his general practitioner (GP) after having some difficulties with his vision. On examination, you find he has a right homonymous hemianopia. Aside from these findings, he is well, although his past medical history reveals that he suffered a transient ischemic attack (TIA) 3 years ago.

Answers

Diagnoses: EMQs

Answer 42

5) Lateral medullary syndrome: Unilateral loss of facial pain and temperature sensation with contralateral loss of pain and temperature sensation of the body is characteristic of the lateral medullary syndrome. This is due to infarction in the territory of the posterior inferior cerebellar artery. Other features include ipsilateral Horner's syndrome and cerebellar signs.

Answer 43

8) Pontine haemorrhage: Haemorrhage into the pons usually occurs as a result of chronic hypertension. Involvement of the reticular formation results in coma. Descending sympathetic fibres cause constricted pupils, and lesions between the red nucleus and vestibular nucleus cause decerebrate posturing.

Answer 44

4) Lacunar infarct of the internal capsule: Lacunar infarcts are due to occlusion or stenosis of small penetrating branches of the middle and posterior cerebral and medial branches of the basilar arteries, usually as a result of hypertension, and cause pure motor or pure sensory loss. They account for approximately a quarter of all ischaemic strokes and have a good prognosis for recovery.

Answer 45

1) Left anterior cerebral artery: The contralateral weakness suggests that the lesion is distal to the anterior communicating artery. The anterior cerebral artery supplies the medial surface and a thin lateral strip of the cerebral hemispheres. The cortical homunculus shows that this area of the primary motor cortex supplies the lower limbs; this explains why the patient's upper limbs are unaffected.

Answer 46

3) Left middle cerebral artery: Most notably, the patient has developed right-sided weakness; this explains his inability to smile properly. A further clue lies in the patient's difficulty with speech comprehension; this suggests he has a lesion in his dominant hemisphere that has caused Wernicke's (receptive) aphasia.

Answer 47

4) **Left posterior cerebral artery**: The homonymous hemianopia (classically with macular sparing) in this patient is strongly suggestive of a contralateral posterior cerebral artery occlusion. Bilateral occlusions of this artery can cause cortical blindness (Anton's syndrome).

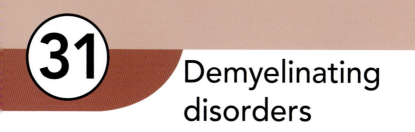

Demyelinating disorders

Questions

Investigations: SBAs

Question 48

A 24-year-old woman presents to her GP with a 1-week history of progressive heaviness and numbness in her right leg. She is referred to the neurology clinic for urgent assessment. When she is seen a week later, the heaviness in her right leg is worse, and examination reveals a brisk knee and ankle jerk and extensor plantar response in the right leg. On closer questioning, she reveals that 1 year ago she had a 4-week episode of blurred vision and pain in her right eye, but it has since returned to normal. Which of the following is the most likely diagnosis? Please choose the single best answer from the following answers:

1) Motor neuron disease
2) Multiple sclerosis (MS)
3) Parkinson's disease
4) Peripheral neuropathy
5) Progressive supranuclear palsy

Question 49

A 35-year-old man has a 6-year history of relapsing and remitting neurological symptoms. During the last 2 years, he has had a 1-month episode of recurrent intense electric-shock-like pain affecting the left side of his face, which eventually stopped with carbamazepine. He recently had an episode of progressive weakness and heaviness in his left leg, and he was unable to walk on it for 2 weeks. The patient is referred to a neurologist for advice on his future management. Which of the following is the most appropriate management? Please choose the single best answer from the following answers:

1) Information and reassurance
2) Interferon 1-beta
3) Long-term oral antibiotics

4) Oral course of high-dose methylprednisolone for 5 days
5) Regular baclofen

Question 50

A 23-year-old woman develops worsening visual loss in her left eye over several days, associated with pain on moving the eye, particularly on looking up. On examination, she has reduced visual acuity in the left eye, and she has lost the perception of colour in the centre of her vision, but the fundi are normal. A swinging torch test shows a left afferent pupillary defect. Over the next 4 weeks, her vision returns to normal. Which of the following is the most likely diagnosis? Please choose the single best answer from the following answers:

1) Amaurosis fugax
2) Giant cell arteritis
3) Occipital lobe lesion
4) Optic neuritis
5) Orbital tumour

Question 51

A 30-year-old woman presents with vertigo, double vision, slurred speech and imbalance on walking. On examination, she has a right-sided dysmetria, brisk tendon reflexes, extensor plantar responses and an ataxic gait. She has a horizontal jerking nystagmus, worse on looking right, and a right internuclear ophthalmoplegia. Two years previously, she had a 4-week period of blurred vision in her left eye. Which investigation is most likely to confirm the diagnosis? Please choose the single best answer from the following answers:

1) Computed tomographic (CT) scan of the head
2) Full blood count
3) Midstream urine sample
4) Magnetic resonance imaging (MRI) scan of the head
5) Visually evoked responses

Question 52

A 48-year-old man presents with a 5- to 7-year history of gradual functional deterioration in his legs. For the last few years, he has noticed that his legs become stiff and heavy if he walks more than a couple of miles, and he has recently fallen over a few times. Over the last few months, he has been having problems with urinary frequency and nocturia. On examination, he has spastic paraparesis with brisk tendon reflexes and extensor plantar responses. Joint position sense is absent in the toes, and touch is reduced up to both knees. There are no eye movement, fundal or cranial nerve abnormalities. Please choose the single best answer from the following answers:

1) Cervical myelopathy
2) Guillain–Barré syndrome
3) Primary progressive MS
4) Relapsing-remitting MS
5) Transverse myelitis

Answers

Investigations: SBAs

Answer 48

2) **Multiple sclerosis**: The history of neurological symptoms affecting the eye 1 year previously followed by upper motor symptoms in one leg is typical of MS.

Answer 49

2) **Interferon 1-beta**: This history suggests two severe episodes of relapsing MS over the last 2 years. Sharp facial pains suggest trigeminal neuralgia, which is a common presentation of MS. Patients with at least two relapses in 2 years often benefit from disease-modifying treatment such as Interferon 1-beta, which has been shown to reduce relapses by 30% in active relapsing-remitting MS.

Answer 50

4) **Optic neuritis**: Subacute unilateral visual loss associated with ocular pain and colour desaturation is typical of optic neuritis. A relative afferent pupillary defect represents damage to the afferent limb of the pupillary light reflex.

Answer 51

4) **MRI scan of the brain**: A previous episode of optic neuritis in combination with the current cerebellar and brainstem features suggests a diagnosis of MS. An MRI scan of the brain would exclude other structural pathology and confirm the diagnosis. A CT scan of the brain may fail to show the white matter abnormalities found in MS.

Answer 52

3) **Primary progressive MS**: A combination of slowly progressive upper motor neuron, sensory and possibly neurological urinary symptoms is typical of primary progressive MS, which tends to affect the spinal cord and is more common in male patients. Transverse myelitis would present more acutely.

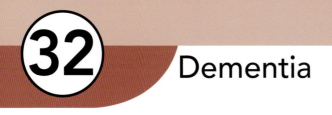

Questions

Diagnoses: EMQs

For each of the following clinical scenarios, choose the most likely diagnosis from the list that follows. Each answer may be used once, more than once or not at all.

Diagnostic options

1) Alzheimer's disease
2) Concussion
3) Delirium
4) Dementia with Lewy bodies
5) Frontotemporal dementia
6) HIV encephalopathy
7) Multisystem atrophy
8) Progressive supranuclear palsy
9) Pseudodementia
10) Vascular dementia

Question 53

A 67-year-old retired postman is brought to his GP by his wife. She is concerned about his change in character over the past 2 years. He is now finding it increasingly difficult to focus on menial tasks. His past medical history reveals two TIAs and one previous stroke, and his wife reports that following each of these there has been a noticeable decline in his everyday functioning.

Question 54

A 72-year-old man is bought to the emergency department in an ambulance after falling and breaking his right radius. On taking a collateral history from his daughter, it becomes apparent that he has become increasingly unsteady on his feet over the past few months, and his memory is poor. On examination, he is bradykinesic, has a unilateral resting tremor, and exhibits a shuffling gait. His Mini-Mental State Examination reveals a score of 20/30.

Question 55

A 76-year-old lady is bought to the hospital after being found by a medical student when the student was on the way home after a night out. The older woman was found wandering in her dressing gown in Sheffield city centre and could not remember how to get home. According to a collateral history from her son, she has become increasingly aggressive over recent months and has on occasion not recognized him when he came to visit. Her Mini-Mental State Examination reveals a score of 19/30, and her physical examination is unremarkable.

Answers

Diagnoses: EMQs

Answer 53

10) Vascular dementia: Vascular dementia is the most likely cause due to his past history of cerebrovascular disease and the classical stepwise deterioration.

Answer 54

4) Dementia with Lewy bodies: The symptoms and signs elicited on history and collateral history are in keeping with parkinsonism and dementia, as seen in dementia with Lewy bodies. These patients can be difficult to manage as drugs used to improve the parkinsonism can cause delusions, and drugs used to treat the delusions can worsen the symptoms of Parkinson's disease.

Answer 55

1) Alzheimer's disease: Patients with Alzheimer's disease are often found wandering or lost due to their problems with spatial navigation and short-term memory.

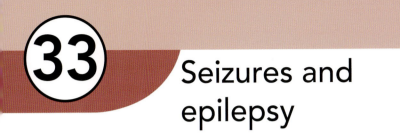

Questions

Diagnoses: EMQs

From the clinical scenarios described, choose the most likely type of seizure. Each answer may be used once, more than once or not at all.

Seizure types

1) Absence seizure
2) Cardiogenic syncope
3) Cerebrovascular event
4) Complex partial seizure
5) Generalised tonic-clonic seizure
6) Myoclonic seizure
7) Non-epileptic attack
8) Postural hypotension
9) Tonic seizure
10) Vasovagal syncope

Question 56

An 18-year-old geography student is taken to the emergency department in an ambulance following her third seizure in a week. She is not known to have epilepsy, and before this episode had never had a seizure. The 'fit' lasted for 35 minutes, and her mother reports shaking of the student's arms and legs. She was not rousable during the attack. She had no obvious injuries and had not been incontinent of urine or bitten her tongue. She had a GCS score of 15/15 on arrival to the emergency department (ED) and was oriented to time and place. She denies memory of the attack. On questioning, she is currently stressed about her exams.

Question 57

A 14-year-old boy is bought to the emergency department by ambulance, accompanied by his panicked mother. About 20 minutes prior, he was playing his new computer game when his mother heard him cry out. She saw him fall from his chair to the floor, his arms and legs stretched out before they started to jerk. She reports that his lips went blue, and he was incontinent of urine. She is unsure how long the seizure lasted, but it had stopped by the time the ambulance crew arrived. He has no history of seizures or other past medical history of note. On arrival to ED, he remains drowsy, and his mother reports that he is 'not with it'.

Question 58

A 32-year-old man is admitted to a neurology ward after he was reported to have had a 'funny episode' earlier this morning. On questioning, his wife reports that he started repetitively smacking his lips and did not respond when she spoke to him. This episode lasted for less than 5 minutes, and then he fell back to sleep. He was well when he awoke later in the morning and had no recollection of the episode. He has no past medical history of note.

Answers

Diagnoses: EMQs

Answer 56

7) Non-epileptic attack: The duration of seizure, quick recovery time, lack of injuries being sustained and no incontinence suggests a non-epileptic attack; however, epilepsy should be ruled out. Patients often find a 'functional disorder' a difficult diagnosis, but given the appropriate counselling, some patients will experience no further seizures.

Answer 57

5) Generalised tonic-clonic seizure: The history is characteristic of a generalised tonic-clonic seizure and should be investigated for a cause. He should also be educated about epilepsy and safety behaviours to avoid any potential injuries. Anticonvulsant therapy is usually initiated following a second seizure.

Answer 58

1) Absence seizure: Unresponsive episodes accompanied by automatisms are suggestive of absence seizures. Typically, they are not associated with abnormal limb movements. As with all new cases of seizure activity, this patient should be investigated thoroughly, and due to the age and denial of previous seizures, this patient should have brain imaging to rule out any structural brain abnormality.

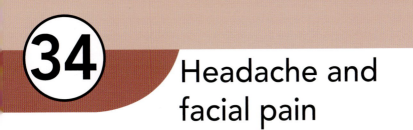

34 Headache and facial pain

Questions

Investigations: SBAs

Question 59

A 43-year-old lady presents to the emergency department with a severe sudden-onset occipital headache. She describes the headache as 10/10 in severity with associated neck stiffness. She also mentions feeling a little drunk. There is no history of fever, and she has not suffered from headaches in the past. What is the most appropriate initial investigation? Please choose the single best answer from the following answers:

1) Blood cultures
2) Clotting screen
3) CT head
4) Lumbar puncture
5) MRI head

Question 60

A 38-year-old teacher presents to her GP with a 4-month history of headaches. She describes the headaches as a tight band around her forehead.
The headaches are worse in the afternoons and exacerbated by stress. There is no neck stiffness, nausea or vomiting, and there is no focal neurological deficit on examination. What is the most likely diagnosis? Please choose the single best answer from the following answers:

1) Cluster headache
2) Migraine
3) Sinusitis
4) Subarachnoid haemorrhage (SAH)
5) Tension headache

Question 61

A 21-year-old television presenter visits the emergency department with a 4-hour history of headache. She complains when the light is on and has vomited three times. On examination, she is drowsy, has neck stiffness, has a non-blanching rash on her legs and is pyrexial. What is the most likely diagnosis? Please choose the single best answer from the following answers:

1) Cluster headache
2) Encephalitis
3) Meningococcal meningitis
4) Migraine
5) SAH

Answers

Investigations: SBAs

Answer 59

3) **CT head**: The history should raise the suspicion of a SAH; therefore, the most appropriate investigation would be a CT head scan. Ten per cent of SAH can be missed on CT head scans, but imaging would be required before doing a lumbar puncture to assess for xanthochromia. MRI is not a first-line investigation in this case, and as there is no fever, blood cultures are unnecessary. A clotting screen would be an appropriate investigation before a lumbar puncture.

Answer 60

5) **Tension headaches**: Chronic generalised headaches occurring in the absence of any red flag features and associated with stress are strongly suggestive of tension headache. Treatment involves reassurance, lifestyle modification and simple analgesia.

Answer 61

3) **Meningococcal meningitis**: Headache, fever and meningism are features of bacterial meningitis. The presence of a purpuric rash is suggestive of meningococcal infection. This is a medical emergency. A lumbar puncture is required to confirm the diagnosis, but antibiotics should be given immediately if this will cause any delay. It is important to obtain senior help as soon as possible and make the high-dependency unit/intensive therapy unit (HDU/ITU) aware of the admission.

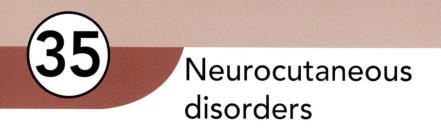

35 Neurocutaneous disorders

Questions

Diagnoses: SBAs

Question 62

A 3-year-old girl is brought into the emergency department by her parents after having a seizure. They say that she suddenly fell to the ground and was unconscious immediately, followed by a couple of minutes of violent generalized shaking. On examination, she is lethargic and has a mild weakness on her right side. She also has a port wine stain on the upper right side of her face. Which of the following is the most appropriate underlying diagnosis? Please choose the single best answer from the following answers:

1) Neurofibromatosis type 1
2) Neurofibromatosis type 2
3) Osler–Weber–Rendu syndrome
4) Sturge–Weber syndrome
5) Tuberous sclerosis

Question 63

A 3-year-old boy is brought to the GP by his mother; the child has a 2-day history of a dry cough, sore throat and raised temperature. Whilst examining him, the GP notices the boy has a red, raised papular rash on his face, shagreen patches on his back and multiple skin tags around his neck. There is also a cluster of hypopigmented confetti lesions on his abdomen. Which of the following is the most appropriate underlying diagnosis? Please choose the single best answer from the following answers:

1) Angiofibroma
2) Neurofibromatosis type 1
3) Sturge–Weber syndrome
4) Tuberous sclerosis
5) Von Hippel–Lindau syndrome

Question 64

A 3-year-old girl is brought to the GP for her MMR (measles-mumps-rubella) booster. Whilst there, her mother says that she is worried about her height as she is much smaller than her peers. She is measured and weighed, and her height is just below the second centile for her age group. On examination, she has seven café-au-lait spots on her trunk, axillary freckles, mild scoliosis and a neurofibroma on her back. Which of the following is the most appropriate underlying diagnosis? Please choose the single best answer from the following answers:

1) Multiple endocrine neoplasia type 1
2) Neurofibromatosis type 1
3) Neurofibromatosis type 2
4) Sturge–Weber syndrome
5) Tuberous sclerosis

Answers

Diagnoses: SBAs

Answer 62

4) **Sturge–Weber syndrome**: A facial port-wine stain is the characteristic cutaneous feature of Sturge–Weber syndrome, which frequently causes seizures due to vascular malformations.

Answer 63

4) **Tuberous sclerosis**: These skin features are characteristic of tuberous sclerosis, in which the main neurological feature is recurrent seizures.

Answer 64

2) **Neurofibromatosis type 1**: Neurofibromatosis type 1 has mainly cutaneous features, including neurofibromata that are often associated with large peripheral nerves.

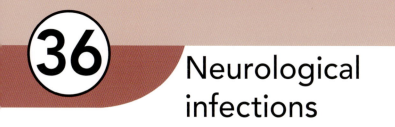

Neurological infections

Questions

Diagnoses: EMQs

Select the most likely causative organism for the clinical scenarios that follow. Each answer may be used once, more than once or not at all.

Causative organisms

1) *Neisseria meningitidis*
2) *Streptococcus pneumoniae*
3) Coxsackie virus
4) *Listeria monocytogenes*
5) *Treponema pallidum*
6) *Mycobacterium tuberculosis*
7) Herpes simplex type 1
8) *Toxoplasma gondii*
9) *Cryptococcus neoformans*
10) *Borriela burgdorferi*

Question 65

A 39-year-old injecting drug user is brought to the emergency department after having a seizure. He has a temperature of 38.7°C and is complaining of a headache, which he says he has had for 5 days. He is confused and has vomited several times. He does not have any neck stiffness or photophobia. A lumbar puncture is performed (after CT scanning), and India ink staining of the cerebrospinal fluid (CSF) shows the presence of encapsulated yeasts.

Question 66

A 19-year-old man originally from Gambia is admitted to the hospital with a GCS of 11/15 and acute onset left-sided facial weakness. His mother attends with him and reports that he has a 3-month history of worsening headache and occasional episodes of fevers and has lost a significant amount of weight recently. CT scanning reveals a communicating hydrocephalus, and the CSF is lymphocytic and has an elevated protein content of 7.4 g/l. No organisms are seen. MRI scanning shows leptomeningeal enhancement.

Question 67

A 30-year-old woman is admitted to the hospital via her GP; she has a 4-day history of flu-like symptoms, including headache and fever. She has mild photophobia and no neck stiffness. CSF analysis reveals lymphocytosis and a mildly raised protein concentration. Her 4-year-old son has recently been ill with a diarrhoeal illness.

Select the most likely diagnosis for each of the clinical scenarios that follow. Each answer may be used once, more than once or not at all.

Diagnostic options

1) Bacterial meningitis
2) Brucellosis
3) Cerebral malaria
4) Herpes simplex virus (HSV) encephalitis
5) Neuroborreliosis
6) Neurosyphilis
7) Primary HIV infection (seroconversion illness)
8) Progressive multifocal leucoencephalopathy
9) Rabies
10) Tuberculous meningitis

Question 68

A 32-year-old man presents to his GP with a week-long history of fevers, myalgia and malaise. He now complains of severe headache and intolerance of bright lights. He has mild neck stiffness. He is admitted to the hospital, where a lumbar puncture shows a lymphocytic CSF with slightly raised protein. He reveals that he has had multiple unprotected sexual contacts with men, the most recent being 8 weeks ago.

Question 69

A 53-year-old woman presents to her GP with a 2-week history of worsening shooting pains affecting both legs and tingling paraesthesia in her feet. She also thinks that the left side of her face has become weak, and she is worried that she has had a stroke. She is a keen hiker, and 5 weeks ago noticed after walking in a forest that a tick had bitten her. A spreading erythematous rash developed at the bite site but has now resolved.

Question 70

A 57-year-old Egyptian man is taken to the emergency department with fever and worsening paralysis of his legs. He can no longer walk. On examination, there is flaccid paralysis of the lower limbs, with remaining power in the hip flexors only. Three weeks ago, he returned from a trip to see his family in Egypt, and he reports that while there he was licked on his feet by stray dogs.

Investigations: SBAs

Question 71

A 70-year-old woman is brought into the emergency department after her son reported her to be markedly confused. She has a temperature of 38.7°C and is complaining of a severe headache and pain in her neck. On examination, she has marked neck stiffness and photophobia. Her son informs the ED staff that she has no allergies, and that she is normally fit and well. A diagnosis of bacterial meningitis is thought most likely. Which of the following is the single most appropriate antibiotic choice? Please choose the single best answer from the following answers:

1) Intramuscular benzylpenicillin
2) Intravenous cefotaxime
3) Intravenous cefotaxime and amoxicillin
4) Intravenous chloramphenicol and vancomycin
5) Oral amoxicillin

Question 72

A 38-year-old man is admitted to the acute admission unit with acute confusion and aggressive behaviour; the background is a 3-day history of headache and fevers. On examination, his GCS is 12/15. A CT brain scan is not immediately available. Which is the single most appropriate action? Please choose the single best answer from the following answers:

1) Administer intravenous cefotaxime and acyclovir
2) Administer intravenous lorazepam sedation
3) Perform a lumbar puncture
4) Perform an HIV test
5) Wait for the results of a CT scan before starting treatment

Question 73

A 35-year-old Pakistani man is brought to the emergency department in a comatose state. His wife reports that he has been suffering from severe headaches for several months and has complained of fevers. Previously, he was fit and well. On examination, he is afebrile, his GCS is 7/15, and he has significant neck stiffness. Fundoscopy reveals severe papilloedema. A CT scan shows hydrocephalus and meningeal thickening. Which of the following is the single most likely diagnosis? Please choose the single best answer from the following answers:

1) Cerebral venous sinus thrombosis
2) Meningococcal meningitis
3) Cerebral toxoplasmosis
4) Tuberculous meningitis
5) Viral encephalitis

Answers

Diagnoses: EMQs

Answer 65

9) *Cryptococcus neoformans:* The presence of yeasts on India ink staining of CSF indicates infection with *Cryptococcus neoformans*. This organism usually causes infection in immunocompromised hosts, although it can also affect the immunocompetent. The typical features of meningism are only rarely seen in cryptococcal meningitis. This patient is an injecting-drug user and is at high risk of HIV infection.

Answer 66

6) *Mycobacterium tuberculosis:* The long history of headache and weight loss in a patient from an area of high TB prevalence is suggestive of tuberculous meningitis. The findings on CT and CSF analysis support this diagnosis. Culture of *Mycobacterium tuberculosis* from the CSF or other sites outside the central nervous system (CNS) is required to confirm the diagnosis. However, clinical features must be relied on when no positive cultures are obtained.

Answer 67

3) **Coxsackie virus**: This lady has symptoms and signs consistent with meningeal inflammation, and the presence of a viral-sounding illness suggests the diagnosis of viral meningitis. An enterovirus such as Coxsackie virus is likely to be the cause.

Answer 68

7) **Primary HIV infection (seroconversion illness)**: This patient has clinical features that are suggestive of meningitis, with a background of a mild systemic illness. Homosexual unprotected intercourse means he is at a high risk for HIV infection. Seroconversion (production of anti-HIV antibodies) occurs within 3 months of exposure to HIV infection and can produce systemic illness as well as aseptic meningitis.

Answer 69

5) **Neuroborreliosis**: This organism (*Borrelia burgdorferi*) is transmitted by ticks in forested and densely vegetated areas, and the initial sign of infection is a spreading erythematous rash at the site of the tick bite: erythema chronica migrans. This lady has features of peripheral neuropathy and cranial nerve palsy (facial weakness), all of which are consistent with neuroborreliosis.

Answer 70

9) Rabies: A history of a bite or other skin contact with mammals in an endemic area should prompt consideration of rabies as a possible diagnosis. This patient has symptomatic paralytic rabies. There is no treatment, and death is inevitable even with intensive care support.

Investigations: SBAs

Answer 71

3) Intravenous cefotaxime and amoxicillin: This elderly lady has all the features of having bacterial meningitis and should be treated with intravenous cefotaxime, but she also requires amoxicillin to cover possible *Listeria* infection. Intramuscular benzylpenicillin could be given in the community prior to transfer to the hospital.

Answer 72

1) Administer intravenous cefotaxime and acyclovir: Viral encephalitis is the most likely diagnosis. However, as CT scanning is not immediately available, administration of appropriate antimicrobial treatment should be given to also cover a possible bacterial infection. A lumbar puncture should not be performed in this patient before the results of a CT head are known.

Answer 73

4) Tuberculous meningitis: Tuberculous meningitis is the most likely diagnosis in a patient from an endemic area who has a chronic headache and fever. This diagnosis is further supported by the CT appearances. Fever and meningism would be unusual in venous sinus thrombosis, and the history is too chronic for bacterial meningitis or viral encephalitis. Toxoplasmosis rarely causes symptomatic infection in immunocompetent individuals.

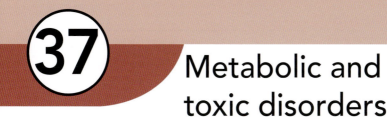

37 Metabolic and toxic disorders

Questions

Diagnoses: SBAs

Question 74

An 86-year-old woman is admitted to the hospital with a community-acquired pneumonia, for which treatment with appropriate antibiotics is started. Over the next few days, she progresses well, and her chest infection appears to be resolving. On the fourth day of admission, she becomes disoriented in time and place and is quite agitated, which her son says has never happened before. Which one of the following is *not* a metabolic cause of acute confusion? Please choose the single best answer from the following answers:

1) Hyperkalaemia
2) Hypernatraemia
3) Hypocalcaemia
4) Hypoglycaemia
5) Hyponatraemia

Question 75

A 40-year-old man who runs a local bar is brought to the emergency department after having a seizure, which was witnessed by his girlfriend. When he is assessed, he is disoriented in time and place and agitated. He is complaining of shaking and headache. He is afebrile, but feels sweaty and is tachycardic. As the casualty officer is talking to him, he says that he can see spiders running all over the floor and walls. Which of the following is the most likely diagnosis? Please choose the single best answer from the following answers:

1) Delirium tremens
2) Opiate intoxication
3) Post-ictal phenomena
4) Viral encephalitis
5) Wernicke's encephalopathy

Management: SBA

Question 76

A 50-year-old man with known cirrhosis secondary to alcohol excess has a large upper gastrointestinal (GI) bleed. He is resuscitated with fluids and made haemodynamically stable. The following day, he becomes increasingly confused and irritable, and a coarse flapping tremor is noted. He is thought to be suffering from hepatic encephalopathy. Which of the following is of use in the management of hepatic encephalopathy? Please choose the single best answer from the following answers:

1) 10% glucose infusion
2) Corticosteroids
3) High-dose intravenous B complex vitamins
4) High-protein diet
5) Non-absorbable antibiotics

Answers

Diagnoses: SBAs

Answer 74

1) **Hyperkalaemia**: All of the metabolic disturbances mentioned may cause an acute confusional state with the exception of hyperkalaemia. A possible explanation for this lady's confusion is hyponatraemia due to the syndrome of inappropriate anti-diuretic hormone secretion (SIADH), which may be caused by pneumonia.

Answer 75

1) **Delirium tremens**: This man runs a bar, which makes him more likely to use alcohol to excess, and the presence of the features of alcohol withdrawal and mental status changes indicates delirium tremens. Wernicke's encephalopathy does not cause hallucination or autonomic symptoms.

Management: SBA

Answer 76

5) **Non-absorbable antibiotics**: Non-absorbable antibiotics are used in hepatic encephalopathy to reduce the production of nitrogenous waste products by gut bacteria. A low-protein diet is also used to reduce nitrogen intake. Corticosteroids are not used in the management of this condition. The B complex vitamins are used in Wernicke's encephalopathy, and glucose is required to treat hypoglycaemia.

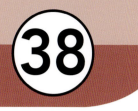

Neurological involvement in systemic diseases

Questions

Diagnoses: EMQs

Select the most likely diagnosis for each of the clinical scenarios that follow. Each answer may be used once, more than once or not at all.

Diagnostic options

1) Behçet's disease
2) Diabetic neuropathy
3) Granulomatosis with polyangitis (Wegener's granulomatosis)
4) Lambert-Eaton myaesthenic syndrome
5) Limbic encephalitis
6) Myaesthenia gravis
7) Sarcoidosis
8) Systemic lupus erythematosus (SLE)
9) Temporal arteritis
10) Viral meningitis

Question 77

A 31-year-old man presents to the emergency department (ED) with a 3-day history of worsening headache and dislike of bright lights. He denies any fevers but reports having a stiff neck for the past day. He attended ED a year previously due to a painful red eye. On examination, there is meningism, and multiple ulcers are noted in the mouth. The patient mentions that he also suffers with ulcers affecting his genital region. A lumbar puncture reveals a lymphocytic CSF.

Question 78

A 64-year-old woman presents to her GP with a sudden painless loss of vision affecting her left eye. She reports that for the past month she has been experiencing an intermittent severe left-sided headache, which she has noticed is worse when she tries to tie her hair back. She also reports malaise and occasional fevers. On examination, she has tenderness over the left temporal region, but fundoscopic examination does not reveal any abnormality.

Question 79

A 27-year-old woman attends her GP with a 4-week history of intermittent generalized headaches. She seems very quiet and becomes tearful when questioned about her mood, which she reveals has been very low recently. She has attended several times over the past year with variable joint pains and has had occasional fevers over this time and felt generally tired. On examination, she has a distinctive rash over the bridge of her nose and cheeks, which she says is worse after going out in bright sunlight.

Answers

Diagnoses: EMQs

Answer 77

1) **Behçet's disease**: This man has presented with features suggestive of meningitis, but there is absence of fever and other systemic illness. The analysis of his CSF confirms aseptic meningitis, for which there are many causes. The history of recurrent oral and genital ulceration and a painful red eye (suggestive of anterior uveitis) would suggest Behçet's disease as the diagnosis.

Answer 78

9) **Temporal arteritis**: This presentation is highly suggestive of temporal arteritis. Monocular visual loss occurs due to anterior ischaemic optic neuropathy, and this complicates around 15% of temporal arteritis. High-dose steroids are required immediately to prevent further visual loss. The contralateral eye can become affected without steroid treatment.

Answer 79

8) **Systemic lupus erythematosus**: This lady has a relatively long history suggestive of systemic illness, with accompanying joint pains and a photosensitive facial rash (butterfly rash). Neurological involvement in SLE can form almost any pattern, but headache is among the most common manifestation. Neuropsychiatric disturbance is also a feature. Stroke can occur and is associated with the presence of lupus anticoagulant and anti-phospholipid syndrome.

Index